CASEBOOK FOR MANAGING MANAGED CARE

A Self-Study Guide for Treatment Planning, Documentation, and Communication

CASEBOOK FOR MANAGING MANAGED CARE

A Self-Study Guide for Treatment Planning, Documentation, and Communication

Jeffrey P. Bjorck, Ph.D.
Janet A. Brown, R.N., C.P.H.Q.
Michael Goodman, M.D.

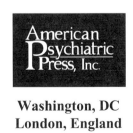

Washington, DC
London, England

Note: The authors have worked to ensure that all information in this book concerning drug dosages, schedules, and routes of administration is accurate as of the time of publication and consistent with standards set by the U.S. Food and Drug Administration and the general medical community. As medical research and practice advance, however, therapeutic standards may change. For this reason and because human and mechanical errors sometimes occur, we recommend that readers follow the advice of a physician who is directly involved in their care or the care of a member of their family.

Books published by the American Psychiatric Press, Inc., represent the views and opinions of the individual authors and do not necessarily represent the policies and opinions of the Press or the American Psychiatric Association.

Copyright © 2000 American Psychiatric Press, Inc.

ALL RIGHTS RESERVED
Manufactured in the United States of America on acid-free paper
03 02 01 00   4 3 2 1
First Edition
American Psychiatric Press, Inc.
1400 K Street, N.W., Washington, DC   20005
www.appi.org

Library of Congress Cataloging-in-Publication Data
Bjorck, Jeffrey P.
    Casebook for managing managed care : a self-study guide for treatment planning, documentation, and communication / Jeffrey P. Bjorck, Janet A. Brown, Michael Goodman.— 1st ed.
        p. cm.
    Companion v. to: Managing managed care II / Michael Goodman, Janet A. Brown,
Pamela H. Deitz. 2nd ed. c1996.
    Includes bibliographical references and index.
    ISBN 0-88048-783-6
        1. Psychiatric disability evaluation—Programmed instruction. 2. Psychiatric
records—Standards—Programmed instruction. 3. Managed mental health
care—Programmed instruction. I. Brown, Janet, 1945– II. Goodman, Michael, 1945–
Managing managed care II. III. Title.
        [DNLM: 1. Mental Disorders—diagnosis—Programmed Instruction. 2. Mental
Disorders—therapy—Programmed Instruction. 3. Forms and Records
Control—methods—Programmed Instruction. 4. Managed Care Programs—Programmed
Instruction. 5. Medical Records—standards—Programmed Instruction. WM 18.2 B626c 2000]
RC470.B58 2000
616.89—dc21

                                                                                    99-040833

British Library Cataloguing in Publication Data
A CIP record is available from the British Library.

In memory of

Michael Goodman, M.D.

(1945–1996)

Contents

About the Authors ix

Preface xi

Acknowledgments xiii

1   Introduction 1

2   The Impairment Inventory: Identifying Impairments 13

3   The Impairment Inventory: Rating Impairment Severity 37

4   The Patient Impairment Profile 71

5   Goals and Objectives: Performance Measures for Managed Care 103

6   The Treatment Plan: Selecting Interventions 131

7   Tracking Patient Progress 149

8   The Discharge Summary: Documenting Treatment Course 169

9   Epilogue..195

Appendix A   DSM-IV Diagnostic Criteria for the Vignette Patients 199

Appendix B   Empirical Research Articles
Patient Impairment Lexicon: A Psychometric Analysis 213
Patient Impairment Lexicon: A Validation Study....................237

References 253

Index 255

About the Authors

Jeffrey P. Bjorck, Ph.D., is an Associate Professor of Psychology at Fuller Theological Seminary's Graduate School of Psychology in Pasadena, California. He is also a licensed clinical psychologist in private practice. Dr. Bjorck obtained his Doctor of Philosophy degree from the University of Delaware, having completed his internship at the University of Oklahoma Health Sciences Center. He has served on the faculty of Fuller Seminary's Graduate School of Psychology for the past 9 years, where his teaching responsibilities include courses in Psychometric Theory, MCMI-III Assessment, Human Learning, and Multimodal Therapy. Dr. Bjorck also conducts empirical research, including the ongoing psychometric evaluation of the Patient Impairment Lexicon, which provides the basis for the Patient Impairment Profile system outlined in this text and its companion, *Managing Managed Care II: A Handbook for Mental Health Professionals* (Goodman et al. 1996).

Janet A. Brown, R.N., C.P.H.Q., is a consultant in quality, utilization, and risk management with psychiatric and medical-surgical, acute and ambulatory healthcare organizations, all of which are now positioning for managed care. Ms. Brown has 22 years of experience in the evaluation, development, and implementation of effective strategies, systems, and processes to meet federal and state regulations, accreditation standards, and review requirements, as well as managed care and employer/payer information needs. Ms. Brown is the author of *The Healthcare Quality Handbook: A Professional Resource and Study Guide,* currently in its 14th edition, and serves as an instructor for quality management professionals preparing for the certification examination. She has chaired the national Healthcare Quality Educational Foundation and was the 1995–1996 president of the National Association for Healthcare Quality.

Michael Goodman, M.D. (1945–1996), was a clinical psychiatrist in private practice in Beverly Hills and Pasadena, California. He attended Tufts Medical School and completed his psychiatry residency at Northwestern University in Chicago, Illinois. Dr. Goodman served for 14 years as a physician adviser with the former California Professional Standards Review Organization and its current successor, California Medical Review, Inc. He was also a consultant in managed mental healthcare with treatment programs and practitioner groups participating in newer managed delivery models. Dr. Goodman was an assistant professor at the UCLA School of Medicine, Department of Psychiatry and Neurobehavioral Sciences, Los Angeles, California. He was also a mental healthcare consultant for the American Medical Association's Doctors Advisory Network, which provides "hands-on" assistance with managed care to members of the American Medical Association. He died on June 17, 1996.

Preface

This casebook is a teaching guide for mental health professionals learning to use the Impairment Lexicon and Patient Impairment Profile (PIP) documentation method. The impairment terminology, PIP, and various treatment plan components (i.e., the "PIP system") provide a "common language" for describing behavior-based patient dysfunction and communicating the clinical rationale for treatment.

The PIP journey actually began before organized behavioral managed care, during a time of increasing concern over rising healthcare costs and the initiation of external review of inpatient mental healthcare. In 1986, the program director of an inpatient adolescent unit, Pamela Deitz, sought consultation on the development of a new quality and utilization management process prior to the unit's first accreditation survey. I was the healthcare quality consultant, and I had a great deal of difficulty tracking the quality and appropriateness of care based on the documentation found in the medical records. A major concern was the multiplicity and variety of goals and behavioral objectives assigned to one patient by each treatment discipline (e.g., nursing, psychiatry, psychology, social work, education). Similarly, assessments and written descriptions of patient behavior associated with a given diagnosis (e.g., major depression) also seemed to vary according to the training and professional orientation of each practitioner on the treatment team.

Michael Goodman, M.D., was the psychiatric director of this same adolescent program. He also was feeling increasingly frustrated, specifically in his efforts to communicate to several new external review organizations the medical necessity and appropriateness of additional hospitalization for the adolescent patients. It became clear that Dr. Goodman and Ms. Deitz's dilemmas both stemmed from the same problem of nonstandardized documentation. We were convinced that there must be a better way to document all aspects of mental health treatment, as well as to communicate with those individuals, groups, and agencies who now need and have the right to know about the treatment. We spent the next 6 years working on the development of a meaningful, serviceable common-language terminology to supplement DSM-IV (American Psychiatric Association 1994). We framed this terminology within the context of a behavior-based documentation system, usable by all mental health professionals who provide patient care and whose services may be subject to review before treatment and/or reimbursement.

The results of these efforts were presented in *Managing Managed Care: A Mental Health Practitioner's Survival Guide* (Goodman et al. 1992). This volume was published at a time of crisis in mental healthcare. Organized managed care—structured as both provider and insurer—began to grow, as did the controls over treatment authorization, selection of treatment delivery setting, and reimbursement. In addition, practitioners and facilities were being asked to apply for preferred provider panels to receive patient referrals.

Soon after the book was published, Dr. Goodman and I approached Jeffrey Bjorck, Ph.D., of the Graduate School of Psychology at Fuller Theological Seminary, Pasadena, California, to conduct independent psychometric research on the Impairment Lexicon and documentation method. First, he and his research team assessed the impairment terminology for content validity to ensure that it comprehensively described all behavior-based patient dysfunctions. The resulting recommendations were the basis for modifications in the impairment terminology incorporated into the second edition of the book, *Managing Managed Care II: A Handbook for Mental Health Professionals* (Goodman et al. 1996). Dr. Bjorck then conducted analogue studies, the first of which evaluated interrater reliability of the Impairment Lexicon. The 20 cases he created for that study became the basis of this casebook. The study also provided recommendations, clarifying some impairment definitions to ensure that they are mutually exclusive. These changes are detailed in Chapter 1 of this casebook and are incorporated into the definitions on the foldout flaps.

Meanwhile, Dr. Goodman and I began to collaborate with a new company, Community Sector Systems (CSS), in Seattle, Washington, to develop software to support practitioners and managed behavioral care organizations. CSS built a computer-based treatment documentation system, using the patient Impairment Lexicon, severity ratings, patient objectives, and practitioner interventions.

Just as the second edition of the book was being released in June 1996, Dr. Goodman died very suddenly. His vision was that every competent mental health professional would have the opportunity to provide high-quality treatment services; communicate patient needs clearly and concisely to all who need to know; document patient impairments, progress, and outcomes well; and subsequently receive reasonable reimbursement. His legacy is the behavior-based common language of impairments and documentation system we developed in this casebook. Dr. Bjorck has facilitated the fulfillment of Dr. Goodman's vision in providing the training method and materials in the casebook.

We enthusiastically pass on to you our passion for clearly articulated, well-documented, skillfully provided behavioral healthcare that can be measured, summarized, aggregated, assessed, and ultimately improved. In an environment that is now quite competitive, with managed care referrals increasingly performance-based, we believe the PIP system offers a way to prove the value of what competent clinicians provide patients: cost-effective quality care with good outcomes. We wish you well.

— Janet A. Brown, R.N., C.P.H.Q.

Acknowledgments

We wish to thank those who helped to make this current volume a reality. First and foremost, our thanks are extended to our colleague, Michael Goodman, M.D., for his boundless energy, enthusiasm, and wisdom. Much of this book is based on his creative contributions to the development of the Patient Impairment Profile (PIP) system. We mourn his untimely death, and we have endeavored to ensure that this casebook reflects his vision for this project.

We acknowledge our appreciation of the editorial staff of the American Psychiatric Press, Inc. (APPI). Specifically, we are indebted to Claire Reinburg, Editorial Director; Pam Harley, Managing Editor; and Carol Nadelson, M.D., Editor-in-Chief, for their valuable assistance with the production of this book. We are also grateful to those formerly at Community Sector Systems (CSS) for the development of software that automates the PIP system. In addition, CSS helped to fund the initial psychometric research with the Impairment Lexicon. Without this research, many of the improvements made in the Lexicon—also featured in *Managing Managed Care II: A Handbook for Mental Health Professionals,* 2nd Edition (Goodman et al. 1996)—would not have been possible.

We also appreciate the excellent efforts of Lisa L. Klewicki, Ph.D., and Christopher A. Leucht, Ph.D., recent graduates of Fuller Seminary's Graduate School of Psychology and student members of Dr. Bjorck's research team. Drs. Klewicki and Leucht made primary contributions to the initial psychometric studies of the Impairment Lexicon, and they also assisted in the development of earlier versions of the 20 fictitious case vignettes presented in this volume. Our thanks also go to Aeri Yi, Linda Rojas, and Chheng Ear for their outstanding secretarial support.

We thank our patients for persevering with us in the ongoing endeavor to reduce the problematic features of managed care and to maximize its positive aspects in the promotion of mental health. Please note that, to protect confidentiality and anonymity, no case depicted in this book represents any real individuals. Rather, these vignettes are based on our collective experiences with patients. Thus, if the names of persons or clinical presentations in this casebook bear any resemblance to real individuals, the similarity is purely coincidental.

Formal acknowledgment goes to James D. Guy, Ph.D., Dean of Fuller Seminary's Graduate School of Psychology, and to Winston E. Gooden, Ph.D., Associate Dean, for their generous provision of sabbatical time to Dr. Bjorck. Without this sabbatical, the current volume would not have been completed. Special thanks are also extended to Daniel T. Suzuki, M.D., Partner at San Marino Psychiatric Associates in San Marino, California. Dr. Suzuki graciously offered his psychopharmacological expertise to support our development of realistic case vignettes.

Finally, and most important, we express our deepest gratitude to our families for their constant encouragement as we completed this project. Special thanks go to our spouses, Sharon M. Bjorck, M.A., and Warren S. Brown, Ph.D., for their continual love, patience, and support.

Introduction

This chapter begins with an overview of the Patient Impairment Profile (PIP) communication and documentation method, described at length in Managing Managed Care II: A Handbook for Mental Health Professionals *(Goodman et al. 1996). The current summary provides a rationale for a new way to articulate and document mental (or behavioral) healthcare. This strategy is not a new assessment or intervention technique. Rather, it is a systematic methodology for justifying why a patient needs treatment now, using behaviorally based, common-language descriptors of current patient dysfunction.*

An outline of the organization of this casebook follows the overview. Finally, updated definitions—based on preliminary research findings—are presented.

Managing Managed Care: An Overview

Managed care can be broadly defined as any patient care that is not determined solely by its provider. Providers of mental healthcare services already are, or soon will be, dealing with managed care systems. The high cost of "unmanaged" care is forcing purchasers of care—employers, insurers, union-management trust funds, and the Medicare and Medicaid programs—to invest in managed mental and behavioral healthcare services. The management of care may include annual and/or lifetime benefit coverage limits, based on the level of care; day, visit, or dollar limits; and limits on the type of disorder or treatment covered or the provider who can be used. Management also may include negotiation of reimbursement rates and methods of payment, preauthorization of treatment (prior to delivery), concurrent review of utilization of services (during delivery), and individual case management.

As the controls in managed care grow, marketplace consumers are pressuring for more healthcare knowledge and more accountability from providers (Barlow 1996). This transformation of healthcare information and services from "private practice" to the public domain is a primary reason that payers, managers, and consumers of care now want performance data—data about the effectiveness and cost of care rendered by both individual practitioners and organizations. Data that are determined to be accurate and are appropriately analyzed and interpreted become valuable information in decision making to a variety of stakeholders (F. L. Newman and Tejeda 1996). Such stakeholders include healthcare purchasers, who develop future contracts; care managers, who select providers and make referrals; and providers themselves, who wish to evaluate and improve their own performance (Howard et al. 1996).

First, providers certainly must attain and maintain their expertise and effectiveness in delivering mental health treatment services. Second, they must become adept at successfully communicating the clinical rationale for these services. Third, they must document services in a systematic way that will provide data about the process and results (i.e., outcome) of care (Chrisman et al. 1996). In managed care, the intention of reviewers or case managers is not to doubt the clinician's expertise or capacity to make good clinical decisions. Rather, reviewers and case managers need to know the rationale for recommended treatments and the supportive, convincing clinical evidence that is the basis for treatment decisions. They want to know why treatment is necessary, why a particular treatment setting or frequency of service is required, and why alternative treatments are not considered appropriate. Mental health professionals must articulate what they are doing for their patients and why they are doing it, or purchasers will be increasingly unwilling to pay for behavioral health services.

This casebook is a teaching tool for the standardized treatment documentation method proposed and detailed in its companion text, *Managing Managed Care II: A Handbook for Mental Health Professionals*, Second Edition (Goodman et al. 1996). This methodology addresses current regulatory and accreditation requirements for clinical record keeping. It also yields efficacious clinical data for measurement of outcomes, research, and the development of practice guidelines. Furthermore, this methodology is being incorporated as the clinical component of communications software for behavioral health applications. It enables the user to perform all the steps required to produce a complete treatment plan and clinical treatment record and contains all the data customarily requested by reviewers for authorization of treatment services.

The purposes of this casebook are threefold: 1) to introduce a behavior-based treatment terminology (outlined below) for efficiently and effectively responding to managed care's need to know about recommended and delivered patient care, 2) to teach—step by step—the communication and documentation method by using this terminology, and 3) to encourage providers to become successful, proactive participants in managed care.

Behavior-Based Treatment Terminology

Behavioral managed care organizations, charged with collecting and interpreting patient and provider data and information to authorize treatment, have varied purposes and business plans and represent diverse interest groups. In addition, reviewers and case managers have widely varied mental health clinical backgrounds. To further complicate the problem, managed care organizations use far from uniform utilization criteria and quality standards or performance measures (R. Newman 1996). Because providers also have multiple levels of clinical training and expertise, the ways in which mental health terms are used in both verbal and written communication are affected.

For these reasons, a common nomenclature for clinical data elements that is readily understood by all parties is desperately needed. Ideally, this terminology would clearly communicate both the reasons for treatment and the thought process—the clinical rationale—concerning the proposed treatment services. The DSM-IV (American Psychiatric Association 1994) diagnosis describes the disorder the patient has and is the conclusive evidence of the provider's ability to synthesize findings (see also Chapter 2). However, DSM-IV cautions, "To formulate an adequate treatment plan, the clinician will invariably require considerable additional information about the person being evaluated beyond that required to make a DSM-IV diagnosis" (p. xxv). In response to this need for additional information, Goodman et al. (1992, 1996) developed the Patient Impairment Profile (PIP) communication and documentation method, described at length in *Managing Managed Care II: A Handbook for Mental Health Professionals*, Second Edition (Goodman et al. 1996).

As a companion text, the *Casebook for Managing Managed Care: A Self-Study Guide for Treatment Planning, Documentation, and Communication* offers an easy-to-use, step-by-step approach to learn the PIP methodology, with particular attention given to the concept of patient impairments. The common-language impairments describe the specific manifestations of the DSM-IV diagnosis, given that it is the manifestations that will become the focus of treatment. *Impairments* are behavior-based descriptors of patient dysfunction. They primarily describe those behavioral dysfunctions for which a person appropriately seeks mental health services. Impairments secondarily identify those conditions that may affect treatment, even though they are not themselves treatment foci. (*All impairments and their respective definitions are listed on the foldout flaps located inside the covers of this casebook.*)

Although impairments are the potential reasons that a patient requires treatment, they are not the reasons for the presence of the disorder, nor are they the disorder itself. Rather, they are observable, objectifiable manifestations that necessitate and justify care, based on the patient's behaviors (i.e., statements and/or actions). There are 64 identified impairments that describe a worsened, lessened, weakened, damaged, or reduced ability to function and, in turn, anticipate a potential for repair, improvement, enhancement, and strengthening of that ability.

Impairments replace "patient problems," those cafeteria-style lists of nonstandardized terms that often fail to communicate not only why treatment is necessary at present but also why it is needed in a specific setting. Lengthy problem lists, in fact, may raise "red flags," signaling that one or more problems are chronic or static (i.e., not treatable). In contrast, the PIP system's identification of impairments is focused on what dysfunctions need treatment now. This information is communicated via the PIP (see Chapter 4*).*

To create a PIP, the clinician often finds it helpful first to compile an Impairment Inventory, which is simply the complete listing of identified impairments. This inventory (see Chapter 2) uses the impairment terminology to identify all cognitive, affective, and behavioral disturbances manifested by the patient during the initial assessment. As such, the inventory becomes part of the assessment. The PIP is created by selecting from the inventory only those impairments targeted for "repair."

Specifically, the PIP will include those impairments that 1) most convincingly describe why the patient needs treatment now and 2) will be the focus of the clinician's treatment interventions.

Communication and Documentation Method

The PIP communication and documentation method addresses current regulatory and accreditation requirements, answers managed care treatment questions, creates a common language to describe patient dysfunction, and standardizes data elements for tracking patient progress and outcome. This method is, in fact, a treatment planning model, informed by the results of assessment and diagnosis. This model assumes that a complete patient treatment plan documents any and all changes over time in the

- Impairments (as noted in the PIP)
- Severity ratings (or severities; as noted in the PIP)
- Treatment goals
- Patient objectives
- Practitioner interventions
- Discharge plan

As previously stated, the PIP—composed of impairments and their severities—provides the framework or focus of treatment. **Impairments,** once identified as the behaviorally based reasons for treatment, establish treatment *necessity*. Next, the recommended treatment must be justified as *appropriate*, a cardinal concern for purchasers of care. Care is appropriate when it is relevant to the patient's clinical needs and consistent with the current state of knowledge and when the benefits outweigh the risks and cost. To establish appropriateness, the clinician must address two questions: 1) How serious is the patient's dysfunction? and 2) What will the patient say or do to show that the treatment is working?

The clinician must assess the seriousness or severity—the extent of dysfunction—of each identified patient impairment. The nature, seriousness, and extent of the patient's difficulties are conveyed as part of the clinical rationale for the recommended treatment. In the PIP method, a **severity rating** is a description of the degree of 1) danger or risk to self or others or 2) compromised function caused by an impairment. Severity is documented with a 5-point scale: 4 = imminently dangerous, 3 = severely incapacitating, 2 = destabilizing, 1 = distressing, and 0 = absent. (*The specific definitions for these five respective ratings are listed in Chapter 3 and on the foldout flaps inside the covers of this casebook.*)

Severity ratings refer directly to impairments—not to the patient who is manifesting these impairments. All of the impairments potentially may be "distressing" or "destabilizing" for the patient (severity of 1 or 2). However, only a certain subgroup of the impairments have the potential to become "severely incapacitating" or "imminently dangerous" (severity of 3 or 4), thereby justifying more intensive interventions. These latter impairments are termed *critical impairments* and are often accompanied by one or more noncritical impairments that affect treatment (see Chapter 3 and the foldout flaps inside the covers of this casebook). In any given patient, the most severe impairment usually determines the most appropriate treatment setting.

Severity ratings must be corroborated by convincing evidence in order to be useful in determining the intensity, frequency, and location of service. The most supportive evidence is that provided by, and described in terms of, patient behaviors—specifically what the patient says (statements) and/or does (actions). The mental health professional must use observation, expertise, and experience

Introduction 5

to identify those patient behaviors that justify decisions about diagnosis, impairments, and related severity ratings.

Once impairments and severities are specified in the PIP, the practitioner's next step is to describe the expectations for treatment. In the PIP method, **treatment goals** logically follow from the PIP, in which one goal is associated with each documented impairment (see Chapter 5). In each case, the treatment goal will be the *repair of the impairment or reduction in severity of the impairment to a treatment endpoint.* The practitioner then lists **patient objectives,** which are *anticipated patient statements or actions that show progress toward repair of an impairment.* As such, objectives also can be thought of as the expected benefits or outcomes of treatment en route to accomplishing treatment goals (see Chapter 5).

After identifying goals and objectives, the practitioner has a sound basis for selecting interventions (see Chapter 6). **Interventions** are *actions taken by a trained mental health professional to modify, resolve, or stabilize the patient's impairments.* Not only goals and objectives but also the clinician's theoretical orientation, experience, and level of expertise will inform the choice of interventions. In addition, the patient's individual characteristics (e.g., age, gender, cultural affiliation, level of religiousness, personal history) must be considered. Therefore, the clinician's expertise is the ultimate "decision rule" for intervention selection. Still, by linking interventions to goals and objectives (and thus also to impairments and severities), the PIP system facilitates both the focus of and the rationale for treatment.

The PIP method and resulting comprehensive treatment plan are dynamic. An ongoing quantified measurement of patient progress is included via documentation of 1) the reduction in impairment severities in conjunction with treatment goals and 2) the percentage of improvement or progress regarding specific objectives (see Chapter 7). The treatment plan provides evidence that treatment is having a positive effect (via documented progress), and it can also communicate the need for continued treatment of remaining impairments. As stated earlier in this chapter, the PIP system proposes that both of these aims are to be accomplished by documenting patient behaviors (i.e., statements and actions).

Finally, a complete treatment plan also incorporates a **discharge plan,** and the practitioner should begin discharge planning at treatment onset. Doing so promotes the view that patient care is a continuum, extending into the realm of self-care following treatment (see Chapter 8). The PIP system encourages the identification of objectives focused on aftercare for every identified impairment. For example, for any given impairment, the following objective can be documented: "The patient will develop a completed self-care plan, including steps to be taken should the impairment return or worsen." By incorporating discharge planning objectives into the treatment plan, the clinician empowers the patient to take ultimate responsibility for self-care during treatment and after treatment completion.

Frequently Asked Questions

Given that the PIP system and its nomenclature (see the "Impairment Lexicon" on the foldout flaps inside the covers of this casebook) are designed to address concerns already described in other ways (e.g., diagnosis, medical terminology), areas of potential overlap can give rise to some questions. What follows is a sampling of questions that we have encountered when introducing the PIP system to mental health practitioners.

Question: *To what extent does the PIP system correspond to DSM-IV diagnostic criteria and a psychiatric style of evaluation?*

Answer: The PIP system and the DSM-IV diagnostic system do *not* correspond; rather, they are complementary but independent. When communicating with managed care organizations, practitioners must answer not only "What is the diagnosis?" but also "Why is treatment needed?" As stated in Chapter 3 of this casebook, 20 patients with an identical diagnosis (e.g., major depression) could potentially have at least 20 different reasons for treatment. Thus, although the PIP system does not correspond to DSM-IV, it is used most efficaciously in conjunction with it.

Similarly, the PIP is not intended to correspond to a psychiatric (or any other) style of evaluation. The PIP is not an evaluation tool but rather is a *communication* tool. It is designed to communicate the practitioner's evaluation results, regardless of what type of evaluation (e.g., psychiatric, behavioral) is selected.

Question: *Most impairment terms in the PIP system appear to be unquestionably linked to dysfunction, but some are not. For example, could someone be an emotional abuse victim without automatically showing impairment and a resultant need for treatment? Could running away represent an adaptive response (e.g., to a physically abusive home)?*

Answer: Being the victim of emotional abuse does not automatically dictate mental health impairment. Unless such victimization results in impairment, it is not appropriate to cite the impairment Emotional Abuse Victim. The same holds true for all impairment terms. For example, running away would not be cited as an impairment if it represented adaptive functioning. (In such circumstances, it might be cited as behavioral evidence for another impairment such as Physical Abuse Victim.) Thus, all impairments are always linked to the presence of mental health dysfunction. Furthermore, all impairments *assume* potential treatability.

Question: *When citing Family Dysfunction or Marital/Relationship Dysfunction, is the "patient" one person or a system of persons?*

Answer: Managed care systems currently are based on the premise of one identified patient per record. Clearly, it is feasible that a clinician might seek to document individual PIPs for several members of the same family system. Whereas some managed care organizations might make provision for multiple identified patients within the same chart, it is more likely that each patient would be identified separately. This would not preclude their being treated conjointly for "shared" impairments (e.g.,

Introduction 7

in family therapy for Family Dysfunction). Conversely, whereas all PIP impairments describe one person, many of them (e.g., School Avoidance, Oppositionalism) might readily suggest conjoint treatment models.

Question: *Why do some impairments appear to describe personality traits (e.g., Egocentricity) when characterological concerns are often viewed as untreatable?*

Answer: The word *egocentricity* might evoke the concept of character traits (and/or Axis II diagnoses). The impairment Egocentricity is not defined as a character trait, however, but as a potentially treatable behavioral tendency existing on a continuum from slight to severe.

When creating the Impairment Lexicon, we attempted to avoid incorporating terminology already commonly used within the mental health profession. This was impractical in some instances, however. *Thus, clinicians must strictly adhere to every impairment term's operational definition to ensure reliable and valid use of the PIP system.* It is never safe to assume knowledge of an impairment definition.

Question: *Some impairment terms appear to overlap. For example, how do Delusions differ from Psychotic Thought/Behavior?*

Answer: Strict adherence to each impairment's operational definition will reveal that no two impairments overlap. Whereas common usage of the term *delusions* could certainly place it within the realm of psychotic thoughts, having delusions without psychosis is also possible. Thus, the separation of Delusions and Psychotic Thought/Behavior in the Impairment Lexicon is necessary because one can have both impairments, one or the other, or neither. Whereas constant reference to operational definitions can appear cumbersome initially, mastery quickly and efficiently provides for reliable universal communication among clinicians, case reviewers, and other relevant parties.

Question: *How does the PIP system address contextual factors (e.g., environmental issues, patient intellectual functioning) with respect to patient assessment?*

Answer: Although contextual factors must be considered when conducting patient assessments, the PIP system is *not* an assessment tool. As stated earlier in this chapter, it is a *communication* tool for conveying assessment results (i.e., reasons for treatment) to managed care organizations. As such, the PIP system assumes that the specific nature of mental health assessments should remain the domain of mental health experts. To the extent that contextual factors provide support for the practitioner's conclusions, they can be cited as evidence for identified impairments.

Question: *The PIP system specifically addresses goals, objectives, and interventions. How are these three concepts differentiated?*

Answer: The PIP system avoids potential overlap among goals, objectives, and interventions in the same manner that it addresses any potential confusion caused by overlapping impairment terms (e.g., Delusions and Psychotic Thought/Behavior, discussed in an earlier answer). In both cases, adherence to strict operational definitions ensures that concepts will consistently remain distinct from one another. Goodman et al. (1996) clearly illustrated the need for such guidelines. They surveyed 156 licensed clinical mental health professionals and managed care reviewers who were asked to label each of 20 statements (e.g., "Implement a no-suicide contract") as either a goal, an objective, or an intervention. (These 20 statements had been obtained from actual treatment records, which supports their content validity for this survey.) Consensus was low, with the experts generally being divided into equal thirds regarding the label for each statement. For example, the "no-suicide contract" statement was labeled as a goal, an objective, and an intervention by 38%, 24%, and 38% of the experts, respectively (p. 113). These results indicate the need for operationally defined terminology in managed care communication. Although adherence to such strict standards might appear cumbersome initially, it is an essential prerequisite for reliable and valid communication.

Organization of This Casebook

General Outline

This book is designed as a self-paced tutorial study guide. Its primary purpose is to provide exposure to the PIP system, with particular focus on the impairment nomenclature. The text is framed around the presentation of 20 case vignettes, each of which depicts an intake interview with an identified patient. Each patient is described as presenting with *no more than 5 impairments*. Together, however, these 20 patients provide examples of every impairment in the PIP system. Thus, the clinician will be exposed to all possible impairments by simply reviewing these 20 cases. In contrast, one would most likely need to see hundreds—if not thousands—of patients to use the entire PIP system in everyday practice.

To facilitate the comprehension of material, each chapter begins with a summary. Chapter summaries are followed by operational definitions of significant terms, initially presented in *Managing Managed Care II: A Handbook for Mental Health Professionals*, Second Edition (Goodman et al. 1996). These significant terms are italicized the first time they occur in the text to signal the reader to their importance.

The chapters provide a sequential exposure to every component of treatment planning, as guided by the PIP system. In Chapter 2, five case vignettes are presented, providing initial exposure to the impairments. The training exercises in this chapter consist of developing an Impairment Inventory for each patient presented. In Chapter 3, five new cases provide the opportunity to refine Impairment Inventory skills. Specifically, the training exercises involve not only identifying impairments but also providing severity ratings for those impairments. The next five cases (Chapter 4) each require the clinician to use an Impairment Inventory as the basis for creating a PIP, identifying those impairments that will be the focus of treatment. Two of these five cases are then revisited in each of the remaining chapters to show how the PIP is integrated with goals and objectives (Chapter 5), interventions

Introduction

(Chapter 6), documentation of progress (Chapter 7), and treatment completion (Chapter 8). These latter chapters also present new cases—two in Chapter 5 and one in each of Chapters 6, 7, and 8. These final five cases permit the clinician to integrate PIP development skills with those facets of treatment planning presented in Chapters 5 through 8. In summary, the seven steps of the PIP system are as follows:

1. The Impairment Inventory is initiated by identifying all of the patient's impairments (Chapter 2).
2. The Impairment Inventory is completed by assigning severity ratings to all identified impairments (Chapter 3).
3. The PIP is created by identifying and prioritizing those impairments from the Impairment Inventory that will be the focus of treatment (Chapter 4).
4. Treatment goals and patient objectives are identified for each impairment in the PIP (Chapter 5).
5. Interventions are selected to treat each impairment in the PIP (Chapter 6).
6. Patient progress is tracked by documenting changes in impairment severities and progress toward meeting patient objectives (Chapter 7).
7. The entire course of treatment, including changes in impairment severities and progress toward meeting patient objectives, is documented in a discharge summary (Chapter 8).

Because the PIP system is intended to complement the DSM-IV diagnostic system, a diagnosis is provided for each identified patient. In addition, the criteria on which each of these 20 diagnoses was based are provided in Appendix A to facilitate understanding of the diagnostic decisions presented.

How to Use This Casebook

This tutorial study guide is designed to provide the clinician with an optimal range of learning strategies. For the individual wishing to master the material most thoroughly, a simple sequential progression through the entire text—with the completion of all exercises—is recommended. Those wishing to focus first on becoming acquainted with the entire range of impairments can do so by simply completing the PIP exercises for the 20 cases presented throughout the book. Conversely, focusing on the explanatory text in each chapter (and initially ignoring the training exercises) is recommended for those who first want to obtain an overall understanding of the PIP system's application to comprehensive treatment planning.

When completing the training exercises, the clinician should note that the correctness of the answers provided can always be questioned. However, initial research on the PIP system that used earlier versions of this casebook's 20 vignettes reported moderate to excellent reliability of the impairments (Klewicki et al. 1998). This same research provided the basis for all *common errors* listed in the text. Still, room for improvement remains, and suggestions for alternative responses to those given in this book are welcome.[1]

---

[1]Please address any such correspondence to Jeffrey P. Bjorck, Ph.D., Graduate School of Psychology, Fuller Seminary, 180 North Oakland Avenue, Pasadena, CA 91101; or jbjorck@fuller.edu.

Definition Updates

Since the publication of *Managing Managed Care II: A Handbook for Mental Health Professionals*, Second Edition (Goodman et al. 1996), continued research efforts (e.g., Klewicki et al. 1998 and Leucht et al. 1999, both of which are reprinted in Appendix B of this book) have provided empirical bases for modifications of the operational definitions of several impairments. Most of these changes were made to improve the mutual exclusivity of the impairment terms, a prerequisite for acceptable reliability of the PIP system. A description of the changes follows (also see the foldout flaps inside the covers of this casebook).

In *Managing Managed Care II*, the definition for *Delusions* was not explicitly distinguished from definitions for *Hallucinations* or *Psychotic Thought/Behavior*. For the PIP system to be optimally reliable, however, there can be no overlap between impairment definitions. Because these three terms are used interchangeably in everyday clinical use, the specific operational PIP definitions for these three impairments are now mutually distinct from one another.

The definition for *Lying* previously did not specify that "deliberate or uncontrolled falsification" had to be of a repetitive nature to signify impairment. Thus, this impairment theoretically could have been ascribed to any patient who reportedly told one deliberate lie. The definition now includes the qualifier "a repetitive pattern" to distinguish it from lying within the realm of normative behavior.

The definition for *Manic Thought/Behavior* previously was not distinguished from that for *Egocentricity*, even though the former includes reference to behavior with "a grandiose quality" and the latter mentions "excessive self-importance." To avoid confusion, these two definitions are now described as mutually distinct. *Manic Thought/Behavior* also is now defined as being "distinguished from *Motor Hyperactivity*" because the former definition refers to "restlessness," whereas the latter refers to "constantly restless" behavior.

The definitions for *Oppositionalism* and *Tantrums* previously included some potential overlap. Whereas the former referred to "provocative contrariness to adult authority figures," the latter mentioned "dramatic outbursts...in response to frustration." Now these two impairments are defined as being distinguished from each other.

In *Managing Managed Care II*, the definition for *Physical Abuse Victim* included the qualifier "*excludes* [emphasis added] Sexual Trauma Victim." Clearly, however, the same individual could experience both of these impairments simultaneously. This problem was resolved by changing this qualifier to "*as distinguished from* [emphasis added] Sexual Trauma Victim." The definition for *Self-Mutilation* was modified in the same way; it now reads "distinguished from [versus excludes] Suicidal Thought/Behavior."

School Avoidance could have been mislabeled simply as one form of *Anxiety*, because the latter impairment included reference to "a state of uneasiness...or dread." *School Avoidance* does not necessarily involve objectively anxious behavior, however, and may relate more directly to oppositional behavior, for example. Therefore, the definitions for these two impairments now have been qualified as mutually distinct.

Another modification in impairment definitions concerned potential ambiguity between *Uncommunicativeness* and *Alexithymia*. The former mentioned "inability to impart...feelings to others," whereas the latter referred to "inability to label affect states...and communicate them to others." Conceptually, these two impairments are quite different. Whereas the former involves an impairment in communication, the latter primarily involves an impairment in self-awareness. Thus, these two definitions are now described as mutually distinct.

As a final modification of the impairment definitions, the impairment term *Marital/Relationship Dysfunction With Substance Abuse* was deleted. Originally, this term had been included because of

Introduction
11

the potentially unique treatment concerns of managed care organizations for patients experiencing a Marital/Relationship Dysfunction with a substance-abusing partner. Additional theoretical and empirical scrutiny, however, revealed that such a compound impairment term is problematic for several reasons. First, it sets the precedent for creating a multitude of such compound impairment terms (e.g., *Family Dysfunction With Physical Abuse, Marital/Relationship Dysfunction With Emotional Abuse*), resulting in the corruption of the Impairment Lexicon's essential reliability. Second, it incorrectly identifies the locus of a patient's impairment as residing in another individual (e.g., one patient needs treatment because another person is abusing substances). Third, compound impairment terms are likely to be readily confused with a simple combination of their components (e.g., incorrectly assuming that the above-described patient is experiencing both Marital/Relationship Dysfunction and Substance Abuse). Finally, documenting impairments for individuals *other* than the identified patient is more appropriately addressed in one of two ways: 1) by identifying the other person as a second patient with his or her own separate PIP and 2) by citing the other person's impairment as supportive evidence for severity ratings, goals, and objectives for the identified patient.

In addition to impairment definition changes, further scrutiny has resulted in a modified definition of the term *treatment goal* (see Chapter 5). In *Managing Managed Care II,* a treatment goal was defined as

> the repair of an impairment or reduction in severity of an impairment to an endpoint or maintenance level. The anticipated reduction in impairment severity may be an *interim goal* or a *maintenance goal.* (Goodman et al. 1996, p. 169)

It became apparent, however, that including both "maintenance level" and "maintenance goal" within the same definition resulted in confusion. As a result, this definition was modified to increase clarity and provide useful distinctions between *types* of treatment goals. The current definition is

> the repair of an impairment or reduction in severity of an impairment to a treatment endpoint. Attaining *endpoint goals* marks the completion of treatment. Treatment involving transition from one *level of care* to another can include an *interim goal(s)* that signals this transition. For patients requiring intermittent and/or ongoing care, treatment can involve *maintenance goals.*

As can be seen, the current definition more clearly demarcates three subtypes of treatment goals, each having unique applications to treatment plan development.

The preceding definition updates are meant primarily for those practitioners who have already acquainted themselves with *Managing Managed Care II: A Handbook for Mental Health Professionals*, Second Edition (Goodman et al. 1996). Those who are just beginning to survey these materials are encouraged simply to refer to the current definitions of important terms (located at the beginning of each chapter) and impairments (located on the foldout flaps inside the covers of this casebook).

Finally, note that this casebook can be used in several different ways (see earlier discussion), but each method involves moving sequentially through the text. By providing several different ways to use the material, however, it is hoped that this casebook will provide an optimal learning experience for each clinician.

The Impairment Inventory

Identifying Impairments

This chapter introduces the Impairment Inventory via five cases, each depicting an identified patient with a DSM-IV (American Psychiatric Association 1994) diagnosis. Each case provides the clinician with an opportunity to select the appropriate impairments, after which answers with rationales are provided. Common errors are also explained.

Definitions

diagnosis   A decision regarding the nature of a mental disorder (using DSM-IV nomenclature), based on an examination of symptoms.

impairment   A behavior-based descriptor of patient dysfunction.

Impairment Inventory   The complete listing of identified impairments.

Impairment Lexicon   A list of 64 impairment terms, each with a specific operational definition, which together describe every potential mental health dysfunction.

Identifying Impairments   **15**

When communicating with managed care reviewers, clinicians must answer the question, "What is the diagnosis?" DSM-IV is the clear standard for accomplishing this task, but it is not without limitations. For example, DSM-IV attempts to "divide mental disorders into types based on criteria sets with defining features...[but it acknowledges]...there is no assumption that each category...is completely discrete...[or] that all individuals described as having the same mental disorder are alike in all important ways" (p. xxii). The resulting overlap between and within categories reduces the likelihood that all persons using a given term will mean the same thing, decreasing the reliability and validity of this nomenclature. Furthermore, managed care systems require that diagnoses be reported, whereas reviewers are more interested in answering the question, "Why is treatment needed?" This is a logical priority, given that 20 patients with an identical diagnosis (e.g., major depression) could potentially have at least 20 different reasons for treatment.

The *Patient Impairment Profile (PIP)* can effectively communicate why treatment is needed. By definition, every *impairment* in a PIP is a "behavior-based [i.e., based on the patient's statements and actions] descriptor of patient dysfunction" (Goodman et al. 1996, p. 167). Obviously, dysfunction warrants treatment with the goal of restoring healthy function. The importance of clarifying why treatment is needed has been made readily apparent at our PIP training seminars. For example, one training exercise involves asking new PIP users to list all the impairments from the *Impairment Lexicon* that could potentially describe one reason that a person with a diagnosis of major depression needed treatment. Invariably, trainees have collectively cited about half of the 64 impairment terms.

The need to go beyond simple classification of mental disorders when developing treatment plans is also acknowledged in DSM-IV. As noted in Chapter 1, DSM-IV states that "the clinician will invariably require considerable additional information about the person being evaluated" (p. xxv) when determining appropriate goals, objectives, and interventions. The PIP provides a means of communicating this additional information to reviewers. In addition, each impairment term is designed to be discrete, and the resulting lack of overlap between impairments reduces confusion and improves communication.

To construct a PIP, one must first make an *Impairment Inventory,* a simple list of all the impairments currently presented by a patient. These impairments may or may not become treatment foci now or later. To identify treatment foci, however, a list of all impairments must be compiled first.

Step 1: Identifying Impairments

Five case vignettes are presented in this chapter, enabling you to begin using and learning the Impairment Lexicon (see foldout flaps). It lists all the impairment terms alphabetically with their operational definitions. Each case vignette includes a reason for referral, history, clinical presentation, and (where noted) assessment assumptions. For each case, you will identify all present impairments and provide behavioral evidence for each one. While reading the vignettes, imagine that you are actually interviewing the patient. Remember that each vignette has *only one identified* patient. Then complete the Impairment Inventory and compare it with the answers that follow. Note that *all relevant information and symptoms are explicitly included in the vignettes.* Furthermore, *no organic psychiatric symptoms (e.g., due to head injury) are presented in any case.*

Casebook for Managing Managed Care

Case Presentation 1

"Frank"

Reason for Referral

Frank, a 24-year-old Caucasian man, was referred to you for evaluation by a local pastor who brought him to your office. The pastor reported that Frank was found talking to himself, shouting obscenities, and singing hymns loudly in the church sanctuary that day. The pastor reported that Frank was conversant but seemed preoccupied and went on to claim that he was hiding in the church because "demons are after me." Frank's mother was contacted, and she reported that Frank "has been 'off' again for the past 2 weeks." You interview Frank and obtain the following information:

History

Frank reports that he "saw his first shrink" at age 15 years when a school psychologist recommended "counseling" in connection with his "bad grades and general strangeness." He was hospitalized the first time at age 18, and psychiatric medication has been prescribed since then "so the voices don't bother me." He reports that he has "been to the hospital a lot."

Frank received his high school diploma at age 17 but never left home, where he lives with his mother (his father is deceased). He has no really close friends, and his primary social interactions are with his mother and occasionally with other participants at a local day treatment program. He has never held a steady job, and he spends most of his time "watching videos, reading comics, and playing adventure games on my computer."

Clinical Presentation

Frank presents as slightly underweight and disheveled. He has apparently not bathed or used deodorant for some time. He does not seem tense or uneasy, but he does appear irritated and distracted. Still, he is alert and can answer your questions. He does occasionally respond angrily, saying: "I don't have to obey you! I just do what they tell me, Doc." Otherwise, he is generally cooperative. During the interview, he occasionally clasps his hands tightly and begins singing loudly. He also swears periodically, and he occasionally stands in order to see out your window. His speech is somewhat pressured but coherent.

His current complaint is that "demons from the movie I watched last week have been on my case ever since. They want to get me, but my singing scares them. Still, I do what they say. I stay in line, Doc." Frank explains that, so far, the demons "tell me to curse people and say bad words." He also believes that they follow him "in those cars with dark tinted windows." When asked about his hygiene, he responds, "Yeah, I know I should clean up my act. My mom is on me about it lately, too." Finally, Frank reports that he feels much better "since they lowered my dose [medication]."

Assessment Assumptions

No substance abuse is present. All factors not explicitly mentioned above have been ruled out.

> **DSM-IV Axis I diagnosis:** 295.30 Schizophrenia, paranoid type
> **DSM-IV Axis II diagnosis:** None

Identify the impairments on the next page.

Identifying Impairments   **17**

Step 1: Identifying Impairments

Instructions: *List **all the impairments, with behavioral evidence (statements/actions),** that accurately reflect Frank's current functioning on the Impairment Inventory below. List the impairments that refer **only to Frank**. Remember that information **not** mentioned should be assumed to be **nonapplicable** to this patient (e.g., no organic pathology is present). Assume that all symptoms and relevant information are reported in the case description.*

Impairment Inventory
1.
Behavioral evidence:
2.
Behavioral evidence:
3.
Behavioral evidence:
4.
Behavioral evidence:
5.
Behavioral evidence:

Turn the page for Impairment Inventory answers.

<table>
<tr><td colspan="1" align="center">**Impairment Inventory**
(Impairments are listed chronologically as they appear in the vignette.)</td></tr>
</table>

1. Hallucinations

Behavioral evidence: They are unremitting. Regarding the "demons," Frank states, "I do what they say. I stay in line, Doc." He specifies that demons tell him to "curse people and say bad words," and he does so (e.g., by "shouting obscenities" in the church sanctuary).

2. Delusions (Paranoid)

Behavioral evidence: They are unremitting. Frank complains that "demons from the movie I watched last week have been on my case ever since. They want to get me, but my singing scares them." He also believes that they follow him "in those cars with dark tinted windows."

3. Inadequate Healthcare Skills

Behavioral evidence: He has apparently not bathed or used deodorant for some time. When asked about his hygiene, he responds, "Yeah, I know I should clean up my act. My mom is on me about it lately, too."

4. Inadequate Self-Maintenance Skills

Behavioral evidence: He has no really close friends, and his primary social interactions are with his mother and occasionally with other participants at a local day treatment program. He has never held a steady job, and he spends most of his time "watching videos, reading comics, and playing adventure games on my computer."

Common Errors

Psychotic Thought/Behavior: This impairment is not appropriate because Frank's bizarre behaviors are totally described by Hallucinations and Delusions. If he showed *additional* bizarre behaviors (e.g., nondelusional peculiar ideation, loose associations), it would be appropriate to add this impairment to his inventory.

Medical Treatment Noncompliance: Although Frank's symptoms may relate to the possibility that "they lowered [his] dose," the vignette does not report that he has in any way failed to comply with treatment.

Obsessions: Although Frank does have thoughts and urges that "force themselves into consciousness," he does not report experiencing them as "unwelcome" thoughts. In addition, he appears to view them as external and real.

Notes

Turn the page for the next case.

20   **Casebook for Managing Managed Care**

Case Presentation 2
"Shirley"

Reason for Referral

Shirley, a 47-year-old Asian American woman, has come to see you because "I just can't stop washing my hands." She is single, has never been married, and lives alone in a nearby apartment complex. You interview Shirley and obtain the following information:

History

Shirley is a computer technician who enjoys her work and has received favorable evaluations throughout the 8 years at her current position. Although she considers several fellow employees to be her "good friends," and she does attend the occasional work-related social functions, "I've always been somewhat of an introvert." Shirley reports that for the past few months, she has been washing her hands "probably 25 or 30 times a day." She tells you that she is repeatedly troubled by the thought that "I might get AIDS by touching something contaminated." The only way that she can obtain relief and/or stop the intrusive thoughts is to wash her hands repeatedly. These problems began for Shirley 4 months ago when another employee left work on disability "and it turned out he has AIDS." Shirley gradually became preoccupied with her AIDS fears and after some time "found that washing my hands seemed to help." This began slowly but increased as the repetitive thoughts became more frequent. "For all I know, half the office has AIDS. I know it's not likely, but anything is possible, and that's what makes me nuts!" Shirley states, "No matter how hard I try, I just can't get beyond this. I feel like I don't have any control over it."

When you ask for more information about her dread of contracting AIDS, she explains that these thoughts and accompanying distress start "first thing in the morning." They quickly gain intensity unless she washes and dries her hands "five or six times in a row." This puts her at ease for a while, but the thoughts often return "within an hour or two"; her distress then increases again until she washes. The urge to wash is not as strong at home, but "the only time I'm totally okay is when I go to sleep at night with the gloves on." (Because her hands have become so dry and chapped, she is using large amounts of hand cream and wearing gloves to bed.) Shirley states that she is aware that "you supposedly can't get it from just touching things, but washing my hands helps me cope. Still, I know it's crazy, and it's starting to help less and less." Apparently no one at work knows yet, "but someone is bound to find out, or at least ask why my hands are so chapped. I just have to get help!"

Clinical Presentation

Shirley presents as a casually dressed, neatly groomed woman of average height and weight. She sits forward in her chair throughout the interview, wringing her hands frequently, and she appears to be shivering slightly. When you ask if she is cold, she says: "I guess maybe a little, but I think it's more my nerves." She is alert and oriented, and her speech is coherent, but her tone suggests a tense, worried mood. Shirley has above-average intelligence. Her hands are badly chapped, and her fingernails are clipped extremely short. She is very cooperative, and she answers each of your questions in minute detail, being careful to include facts such as times and dates.

Assessment Assumptions

No substance abuse is present. All factors not explicitly mentioned above have been ruled out.

> **DSM-IV Axis I diagnosis:** 300.3 Obsessive-compulsive disorder
> **DSM-IV Axis II diagnosis:** None

Identify the impairments on the next page.

Identifying Impairments

21

Step 1: Identifying Impairments

Instructions: *List **all the impairments, with behavioral evidence (statements/actions),** that accurately reflect Shirley's current functioning on the Impairment Inventory below. List the impairments that refer **only to Shirley**. Remember that information **not** mentioned should be assumed to be **nonapplicable** to this patient (e.g., no organic pathology is present). Assume that all symptoms and relevant information are reported in the case description.*

Impairment Inventory
1.
Behavioral evidence:
2.
Behavioral evidence:
3.
Behavioral evidence:
4.
Behavioral evidence:
5.
Behavioral evidence:

Turn the page for Impairment Inventory answers.

Impairment Inventory
(Impairments are listed chronologically as they appear in the vignette.)

1. Obsessions
Behavioral evidence: She is repeatedly troubled by "the thought that I might get AIDS by touching something contaminated." She feels "like I don't have any control over it." The only way that she can obtain relief and/or stop the intrusive thoughts is to wash her hands repeatedly. "I know it's crazy, and it's starting to help less and less."

2. Compulsions
Behavioral evidence: Shirley says: "I just can't stop washing my hands....probably 25 or 30 times a day." The only way that she can obtain relief and/or stop her intrusive thoughts is to wash and dry her hands five or six times in a row. Washing her hands helps her "cope."

3. Anxiety
Behavioral evidence: Shirley constantly dreads the thought of getting AIDS by touching something contaminated, even though she acknowledges, "I know it's crazy." Still, she is able to control her distress, as "washing my hands helps me cope," and anxiety is apparently not a problem during the night. In session, her frequent hand-wringing, shivering, and speech suggest a tense, worried mood.

Common Errors

Delusions (Nonparanoid):   Shirley does not exhibit "beliefs obviously contrary to demonstrable fact." Rather, regarding her fears and behaviors, she states "I know it's crazy." As such, her fears about the *possibility* of contracting AIDS are not delusional.

Phobia: Shirley's fears are not directly related to either "persons, places, or things." Rather, she experiences anxiety in connection with the unwelcome idea (i.e., obsession) that she might somehow contract AIDS (see "Anxiety" above).

Identifying Impairments

Notes

Turn the page for the next case.

24   Casebook for Managing Managed Care

Case Presentation 3
"Yolanda"

Reason for Referral

Yolanda, a single 24-year-old Latina woman, was referred to you by the Employee Assistance Program at the automobile assembly plant where she works as a heavy machine operator. Yolanda reports having received good evaluations at work until 3 months ago, when her supervisor told her that her productivity was down and that her sick leave time was almost used up. Last week, her supervisor caught her drinking in the rest room. Yolanda admits she has been "a little stressed out lately, but it's nothing I can't handle." She further states that she is "angry they made me see a shrink." You interview Yolanda and obtain the following information:

History

Yolanda reports never having been to counseling before. She received her high school diploma, having earned "Bs and Cs." She then worked as a cashier for 4 years while living at home with her mother and younger brother (her parents were divorced when she was 11 years old). She became an assembly-line worker at the automobile plant 2 years ago; she moved into an apartment with her boyfriend at that time. Yolanda reports that she did well for the first year. Her boyfriend left 6 months ago, however, "because we couldn't deal with each other 24 hours a day. Living together turned out to be a real drag." Only an occasional drinker before the breakup, Yolanda reports that she then began drinking more heavily "especially at night after work, alone in my stupid apartment." She denies any drug use, and her required drug screens at work have all had negative results.

Yolanda reports that she had some good friends during high school, but she lost contact with many of them when she became involved with her former boyfriend. This relationship had been her first (having dated since her senior year), and she has not seriously dated since the breakup. She has tried renewing some friendships "but they're all in relationships, so it's tough for us to get together." Without her boyfriend's income, she reports that "it's been a challenge just to make ends meet and pay the rent." She has also grown tired of her job but does not know if she could find another. She adds, "there's no time to look."

Clinical Presentation

Yolanda presents as a casually dressed, neatly groomed, and slightly overweight woman who appears oriented and coherent. She speaks somewhat slowly with little voice modulation. She also delays at times before responding to questions, and she rarely shifts her position in her chair. She is generally cooperative despite her somewhat angry demeanor. During the interview, eye contact is only intermittent. Initially guarded, she appears more comfortable as the session progresses.

Yolanda acknowledges that she now "might be drinking a bit too much, but it's nothing I can't handle." She explains that her drinking helps her "pass the time" and that she now plans to "cut way down." She states that she never drinks and drives because "I have too much sense to be that stupid," and she admits being embarrassed about being caught at work. Regarding her emotional state, she reports "I feel fine, just bored with my job." She also complains that she has had "recent trouble concentrating on my dumb assembly work." Furthermore, she finds it more difficult to pay attention even to leisure activities. Specifically, she says, "I can't read a book or even watch TV for long, although a drink can help sometimes." She also is aware that she is not working as quickly as she did during her first year of work.

Assessment Assumptions

Substance abuse history does not precede the current situation. All factors not explicitly mentioned above have been ruled out.

> **DSM-IV Axis I diagnosis:** 305.00 Alcohol abuse
> **DSM-IV Axis II diagnosis:** None

Identify the impairments on the next page.

Identifying Impairments   25

Step 1: Identifying Impairments

Instructions: *List **all the impairments, with behavioral evidence (statements/actions),** that accurately reflect Yolanda's current functioning on the Impairment Inventory below. List the impairments that refer **only to Yolanda**. Remember that information **not** mentioned should be assumed to be **nonapplicable** to this patient (e.g., no organic pathology is present). Assume that all symptoms and relevant information are reported in the case description.*

Impairment Inventory
1.
Behavioral evidence:
2.
Behavioral evidence:
3.
Behavioral evidence:
4.
Behavioral evidence:
5.
Behavioral evidence:

Turn the page for Impairment Inventory answers.

<table>
<tr><td colspan="1">**Impairment Inventory**
(Impairments are listed chronologically as they appear in the vignette.)</td></tr>
<tr><td>**1. Substance Abuse**</td></tr>
<tr><td>Behavioral evidence: She is almost "out of sick leave"; her supervisor caught her drinking on the job, where she works with heavy machinery; and she often drinks alone at home to pass the time.</td></tr>
<tr><td>**2. Psychomotor Retardation**</td></tr>
<tr><td>Behavioral evidence: Yolanda's productivity is down at work, her speech is slowed, and her responses are delayed. She seldom shifts once seated.</td></tr>
<tr><td>**3. Decreased Concentration**</td></tr>
<tr><td>Behavioral evidence: Yolanda finds it harder to concentrate at work and also at home, even on leisure activities such as reading or watching TV.</td></tr>
</table>

Common Errors

Dysphoric Mood: Yolanda's presentation might lead many clinicians to conclude that she is experiencing *latent* depressive symptoms, obscured by Substance Abuse. Note, however, that *only current behaviorally supportable impairments are to be listed in an Impairment Inventory.* Currently, Yolanda reports, "I feel fine, just bored with my job." Additionally, she does appear somewhat angry, but she provides no behavioral evidence of "conscious and apparent...sadness, gloominess." Thus, Dysphoric Mood, as defined, is not present. If this impairment does become evident in the future (e.g., as Substance Abuse diminishes), it would then be appropriate to add Dysphoric Mood to the inventory.

Alexithymia: Those clinicians tempted to attribute latent depressive symptomatology to Yolanda might also presume her report of feeling "fine" is due to "impaired ability to label affect states." No behavioral evidence exists for such an impairment, however. Note that impairments do not describe a clinician's *interpretation* of a patient's statements and actions. Rather, they simply describe the statements and actions themselves. Currently, Yolanda reports no difficulty labeling affect states, and her behavior does not support such difficulty.

Social Withdrawal: Although Yolanda is living in relative isolation at present, this is not the result of her own "curtailment or cessation of interpersonal relationships." Rather, she even reports attempts to renew some friendships "but they're all in relationships, so it's tough for us to get together." Thus, her isolation represents a life stressor rather than a behavioral response to stress.

Identifying Impairments

Notes

Turn the page for the next case.

28   Casebook for Managing Managed Care

Case Presentation 4
"Pam"

Reason for Referral

Pam, a 15-year-old Caucasian female, was referred to you by a physician from the local hospital. She was rushed to the emergency room yesterday after she called 911 and reported, "I just took a bunch of Tylenol." Medical examination found no physical danger and supported Pam's claim that she had ingested "about six or eight tablets." Physicians also discovered bruises on her buttocks and thighs, which she attributed to "falling down" recently. You review her chart progress notes from the emergency department and speak with her mother. Then you interview Pam alone and obtain the following information:

History

Pam lives with her mother and 8-year-old sister Denise. Her parents divorced 3 years ago, and both she and her sister spend every other weekend with their father. Currently a high school sophomore, Pam did not have any significant problems until 8 months ago. Then she began to feel that "the guys would only check out the thin girls," and she became preoccupied with losing weight. When dieting failed, she began to self-induce vomiting after lunch at school. At the same time, she began buying "lots of junk food." "Once I started eating, I couldn't stop." Soon, she was doing this "two or three times a week." Afterward, she says, "I would feel guilty, and I'd get rid of it [vomit] to feel better." Her mother works days and has been unaware of Pam's bingeing and purging. "Besides," Pam continues, "I like school and get okay grades, so she probably thinks everything is fine. Anyway, she spends most of her time with Denise when she's not working." When asked about her "overdose," she replies, "I don't know. I guess I'm tired of being so fat and throwing up all the time. I guess it was pretty dumb."

Her mother reports feeling badly "about this whole thing" but says she needs to work a lot to support her family. She states, "I didn't know there was a problem." She also claims that her ex-husband "lets them do whatever they want when they are with him," and this frustrates her. Still, she reports that her daughters have "been good when they're with me at least, and they do fine in school."

When you ask Pam how she could possibly get such bruises by falling down, she reluctantly reports, "Dad got mad at me when I came home late last Friday. He's been getting mad a lot lately." She also reveals that "Dad always says, 'you're a loser just like your mother!' Lately, he either ignores me or just yells. I only go there to see my boyfriend." When you ask why she has said nothing about her physical injuries, she explains that she gets to see her boyfriend (who lives near her father) only during weekends at her dad's house.

Clinical Presentation

Pam presents as an only slightly overweight and casually dressed girl wearing makeup, black jeans, and a rock concert T-shirt. She is calm, coherent, and generally responsive, appearing hesitant only when asked about her bruises. Afterward, she persistently repeats, "Please don't tell my dad." She admits that "I didn't really want to kill myself. I guess I was just pretty mad about everything." She reports enjoying school, her friends, and her boyfriend.

Assessment Assumptions

No sexual abuse or substance abuse is present. All factors not explicitly mentioned above have been ruled out.

> **DSM-IV Axis I diagnosis:** 307.51 Bulimia nervosa
> **DSM-IV Axis II diagnosis:** None

Identify the impairments on the next page.

Identifying Impairments

Step 1: Identifying Impairments

Instructions: *List **all the impairments, with behavioral evidence (statements/actions),** that accurately reflect Pam's current functioning on the Impairment Inventory below. List the impairments that refer **only to Pam**. Remember that information **not** mentioned should be assumed to be **nonapplicable** to this patient (e.g., no organic pathology is present). Assume that all symptoms and relevant information are reported in the case description.*

Impairment Inventory
1.
Behavioral evidence:
2.
Behavioral evidence:
3.
Behavioral evidence:
4.
Behavioral evidence:
5.
Behavioral evidence:

Turn the page for Impairment Inventory answers.

Impairment Inventory
(Impairments are listed chronologically as they appear in the vignette.)

1. Suicidal Thought/Behavior

Behavioral evidence: She took eight Tylenol, but then called 911. She states, "I guess it was dumb…I didn't really want to kill myself. I…was just mad about everything." She enjoys school, her friends, and her boyfriend. She does not appear depressed.

2. Physical Abuse Victim

Behavioral evidence: Physicians discovered bruises. She reports that her father "got mad [and hit her?]." She is currently in the hospital, not staying with her father.

3. Emotional Abuse Victim

Behavioral evidence: She reports that her father has "been getting mad a lot lately…[and that he] always says, 'you're a loser just like your mother!'" She also states that he "either ignores me or just yells."

4. Eating Disorder

Behavioral evidence: Pam is preoccupied with losing weight, including dieting and self-induced vomiting after lunch. She binges on "lots of junk food…to feel better…two or three times a week." Afterward, she feels "guilty" and purges. She took Tylenol because she hates "being so fat and throwing up all the time."

5. Family Dysfunction

Behavioral evidence: Her mother reportedly "didn't know there was a problem" and "spends most of her time with Denise when she's not working." Her mother states that Pam's father "lets them do whatever they want."

Common Errors

Self-Esteem Deficiency: Some clinicians might be tempted to view Pam's suicide attempt as representing "inadequate or absent regard for oneself." Pam states, however, that her attempt "was dumb….I didn't really want to kill myself." Furthermore, she enjoys school, her friends, and her boyfriend. Thus, her suicide attempt appears to represent an impulsive behavior rather than an ongoing "absent regard for oneself."

Medical Risk Factor: Although maintaining an Eating Disorder can create medical risks, medical risk factor *as an impairment* is not present for Pam. Specifically, this impairment involves "any adverse reaction or other medical complication that could result" *from the initiation of certain treatments*. No facet of her treatment is described as entailing such risk.

Identifying Impairments

Notes

Turn the page for the next case.

32   **Casebook for Managing Managed Care**

Case Presentation 5
"George"

Reason for Referral

George, a 40-year-old African American man, was court-referred for "counseling" by a report to the Department of Child Protective Services. Specifically, it was recently reported (and confirmed) that George has been sexually abusing his 10-year-old daughter Samantha ("Sam") during the past year. You interview George, with his wife Michelle and his 17-year-old son David, and obtain the following information:

History

George works as a butcher at a local supermarket, and his wife works part-time as a housekeeper for a cleaning business. His son is in twelfth grade, and his daughter is in fifth grade. After an investigation of complaints she made to a school counselor, Sam was removed from the home by the Department of Child Protective Services 1 month ago and remains in foster care. Once his wife supported their daughter's complaints, George pled guilty to the charges of abuse (although he still denies the severity of the allegations, which include vaginal penetration). His wife states, "I always thought Sam was just lying to get attention, but when the school counselor spoke to me, the pieces all came together for the first time."

When you speak to George's son alone, he claims that he too was fondled sexually by his father until he entered high school. He explains, "I was always too embarrassed to tell Mom. Now that I'm bigger than he is, he just leaves me alone." When you see George's wife alone, she reveals that George rarely has shown interest in a sexual relationship with her for the past 3 years. She reports, "all he does anymore is criticize me and insult me, almost as much as he does to Sam." She continues, "I know it sounds silly, but I think George has always been angry that we had a girl instead of another son. I think that's why he always puts her down." When you ask for clarification, she explains, "He often tells Sam she's no good and that she'll never amount to anything. Sometimes he even calls her 'our little mistake.'" George's wife admits that she has often considered divorcing him, "but we need the two incomes, and I could never leave the kids with him." When you ask her if George has ever physically abused the children, she replies "Oh, never! If he did that, I would have left long ago and taken the kids with me."

Clinical Presentation

George presents as a short, stocky man who is neatly dressed and groomed. He appears irritated throughout the interview and protests being required to "get counseling." When you interview the family together, George and his son David do most of the talking, often speaking over each other. George's wife sits passively next to him and rarely speaks. George accepts the abuse charges but attempts to deny or minimize their severity. When he does so, his wife sighs and shakes her head while David verbally defends his sister.

When you see George alone, he again admits fondling Samantha but still denies engaging in sexual intercourse. When you ask him to explain why the medical examination found that she has experienced vaginal penetration, he replies: "How do I know? She's a dumb enough kid. Maybe she was messing around and did it to herself by accident." George further states, "I don't know why they make such a big deal about touching your own kid. I think this sex abuse stuff in the media has the whole country going crazy over nothing. Besides, I think it's good for kids to learn about sex at home instead of on the streets."

Assessment Assumptions

No substance abuse or physical abuse is present. All factors not explicitly mentioned above have been ruled out.

> **DSM-IV Axis I diagnosis:** 302.2 Pedophilia, sexually attracted to both
> **DSM-IV Axis II diagnosis:** None

Identify the impairments on the next page.

Identifying Impairments

Step 1: Identifying Impairments

Instructions: *List all the impairments, with behavioral evidence (statements/actions), that accurately reflect George's current functioning on the Impairment Inventory below. List the impairments that refer only to George. Remember that information not mentioned should be assumed to be nonapplicable to this patient (e.g., no organic pathology is present). Assume that all symptoms and relevant information are reported in the case description.*

Impairment Inventory
1.
Behavioral evidence:
2.
Behavioral evidence:
3.
Behavioral evidence:
4.
Behavioral evidence:
5.
Behavioral evidence:

Turn the page for Impairment Inventory answers.

Casebook for Managing Managed Care

Impairment Inventory
(Impairments are listed chronologically as they appear in the vignette.)

1. Emotional Abuse Perpetrator

Behavioral evidence: George reportedly often criticizes and insults his wife. He reportedly tells Samantha that she's no good, that she'll never amount to anything, sometimes calling her "our little mistake." George describes Samantha as "a dumb enough kid."

2. Sexual Trauma Perpetrator

Behavioral evidence: George confessed to fondling Samantha, the medical examination confirms vaginal penetration, and George's son David claims that he also was abused in the past. No imminent danger is present, however, because Samantha is out of the home, and David is "bigger than he is."

3. Sexual Object Choice Dysfunction

Behavioral evidence: George has repeatedly chosen his daughter as a sexual object and has allegedly chosen his son in the past. He states, "I don't know why they make such a big deal about touching your own kid....I think it's good for kids to learn about sex at home instead of on the streets."

4. Family Dysfunction

Behavioral evidence: George has grossly violated his daughter's rights (i.e., emotional, sexual), the parents are not a team (mother appears very passive), and George is apparently alienating all family members.

5. Marital/Relationship Dysfunction

Behavioral evidence: George reportedly has shown little sexual interest in Michelle for the past 3 years. Michelle states, "all he does anymore is tell me what he wants done around the house and then he yells that I never do anything right." When interviewed together, George dominates and Michelle rarely speaks and appears passive/dependent.

Common Errors

Lying: George does deny confirmed allegations of having intercourse with his daughter. This one lie, however, does not represent "a repetitive pattern of deliberate or uncontrolled falsification."

Externalization and Blame: This impairment is not present because George accepts his abuse charges and blames no one for them. Thus, his attempts to deny or minimize the charges' severity appear to be motivated by other factors (e.g., a fear of legal repercussions). In contrast, if he had attributed his sexual misconduct to other factors (e.g., seduction by his daughter or unsatisfactory sexual relations with his wife), Externalization and Blame would apply.

Notes

The Impairment Inventory
Rating Impairment Severity

In this chapter, severity ratings are presented as a means for justifying the appropriateness of treatment, and five new cases are presented. As in the previous chapter, each case vignette is followed by an Impairment Inventory exercise with answers. In this chapter, however, the clinician then has the opportunity to assign impairment severity ratings and compare them with provided answers with rationales. Once again, common errors are explained.

Definitions

clinical necessity Verification of the clinical need for appropriate treatment in the appropriate setting as evidenced by the patient's behaviors (statements and actions) and severity ratings.

clinical rationale The relevance of the patient's behaviors to the identified impairments, or the stated behaviors and severity ratings to justify the identified impairments.

critical impairment One of a predetermined subgroup of patient impairments that have the potential to justify a more service-intensive treatment or setting (e.g., hospitalization).

severity rating A description of the degree of 1) danger or risk to self or others or 2) compromised function due to an impairment.

As stated in Chapter 2, the Impairment Inventory is simply a list of identified patient impairments, any of which may or may not be included in the Patient Impairment Profile (PIP). For example, a practitioner would not include an impairment from the Inventory in a PIP unless treatment of that dysfunction was assessed as feasible for that patient. Likewise, a practitioner would not select an impairment for the PIP that might be treated later but not now.

Before creating a PIP, however, the practitioner completes the Impairment Inventory by rating the severity of each listed impairment. For those impairments that will *not* be included in the PIP, *severity ratings* still serve as valuable contextual information. For those impairments that are selected, severity ratings help to address the reviewers' question "*How much* treatment is needed?" in terms of both quantity and intensity of service. By presenting impairments with ratings of their severity, clinicians can provide not only a *clinical rationale* for treatment but also evidence for the treatment's *clinical necessity*. Severity ratings do not, however, automatically dictate the treatment levels of care. Determining appropriate treatment settings still requires the clinician's judgment, in light of all known factors.

A five-point scale is used for rating impairment severity. Numerical information is easily communicated to reviewers and facilitates the tracking of progress. Note, however, that this scale lacks great precision, and judging impairment severity is the clinician's responsibility, based on available data and expertise. The five ratings are as follows:

4   **Imminently dangerous:** predictably destructive to oneself or others, or completely compromises (>90%) self-care functioning.

3   **Severely incapacitating:** potentially/probably dangerous to oneself or others, or severely compromises (61%–90%) self-care functioning.

2   **Destabilizing:** markedly compromises (30%–60%) self-care functioning, or inhibits the effectiveness of treatment or support systems for "repairing" the impairment.

1   **Distressing:** compromises (<30%) self-care functioning, or, although currently absent, impairment potentially/probably could occur/recur without treatment.

0   **Absent:** repaired or nonpathological. (Note: This rating is not used when initially establishing a PIP, but only thereafter to denote progress or outcome regarding identified impairments.)

When using this scale, the clinician must remember that impairment severity ratings *do not describe how upsetting an impairment is* for the patient. Rather, they describe the degree to which the impairment inhibits the patient's level of self-care functioning (i.e., to what extent does the problem impair the patient's functioning?). Preliminary research findings suggest that the former misconception can be common initially.

To illustrate this potential confusion, consider two different patients who both manifest Altered Sleep. One patient reports that she has begun having difficulty falling asleep 2 or 3 nights per week and that this change in her sleeping habits upsets her greatly. Based on her emotional response to this impairment, a clinician might be tempted to rate her Altered Sleep with a severity of 3. Note, however, that the patient's sleep problem inhibits her optimal self-care functioning only in a minor way (and would thus probably be given a severity rating of 1). However, the patient's upset feelings might warrant the citing of an additional impairment, Dysphoric Mood. In contrast, a second patient reports difficulty falling asleep 4 or 5 nights per week, frequent waking, and chronic fatigue, but this patient might claim that his sleep problem is merely a nuisance. Based on the patient's mild distress level, one might assign a severity rating of 1. In this case, however, the Altered Sleep clearly inhibits optimal self-care functioning in a more pronounced way (and would thus probably be given a severity

Rating Impairment Severity
39

rating of 2). The competent clinician would also note this patient's lack of concern about his Altered Sleep as meriting additional exploration in its own right.

As a second example, an Educational Performance Deficit can never impair a patient's functioning beyond a severity rating level of 2. First, this impairment can never cause the patient to be potentially/probably dangerous to oneself or others, nor can it severely compromise (61%–90%) self-care functioning, because much of self-care can be done without any formal education. Clinicians must keep in mind that *severities rate the specific impairments and not the patient.*

Critical Versus Noncritical Impairments

Goodman et al. (1996) theorized that all impairments might be "distressing" or "destabilizing" (i.e., severity of 1 or 2), but only some impairments can be either "severely incapacitating" or "imminently dangerous" (i.e., severity of 3 or 4). These latter impairments are classified (and denoted on the foldout flaps) as *critical,* because they may warrant more intensive treatment (e.g., hospitalization). Thus, by definition, *noncritical* impairments alone (e.g., Altered Sleep) typically will not provide a clinical rationale for such service intensity. Some clinicians might be tempted to rate a noncritical impairment with a severity of 3 or 4. In such cases, the patient most likely has a critical impairment (e.g., Dysphoric Mood) *in addition to* a noncritical impairment. Clearly, it is important for clinicians to document *all* impairments, which can have interactive implications for treatment. Conversely, clinicians should avoid "stuffing" inventories in an attempt to justify treatment. Treatment authorization will more likely be based on the impairment with the highest rating than on the simple number of impairments.

Step 2: Rating Impairment Severity

Five new case vignettes are presented in this chapter. As in Chapter 2, you will use the Impairment Lexicon (see foldout flaps) to identify impairments and then provide behavioral evidence for each one. Then, you will also rate each impairment's severity (see foldout flaps for ratings) and provide a behavioral (statement/action) rationale for your ratings. Please note that your behavioral evidence for impairments and your severity rationale for their severity ratings *may overlap or be identical,* because the same information often can be used for both purposes. As in Chapter 2, please read the vignette and imagine that you are actually interviewing the patient. Then complete the Impairment Inventory, and compare it with the answers that follow.

Case Presentation 6
"Mark"

Reason for Referral

Mark, a 29-year-old Asian American man, was referred to you by his physician because of difficulty maintaining an erection. His physician ruled out physical causes and then suggested that "marriage counseling" might help. Mark scheduled the appointment with you and asked that his wife, Susan, a 31-year-old Asian American woman, come with him. You interview Mark and Susan, together and separately, and obtain the following information:

History

Mark and Susan have been married 5 years. Mark is a paralegal, and Susan is a laboratory technician. When you see them together, only Susan answers while Mark is generally silent. She states, "our marriage was pretty good for the first 3 years, but then Mark began to 'pull away' from me. He started sharing less about his feelings, and he'd often say, 'I don't know' to my questions. Lately, he hardly talks to me. It's just not like him! He's the sweetest guy I've ever known." Susan further reports that their sex life was okay until 4 months ago when Mark began having problems maintaining an erection. During the last two attempts, which both occurred 3 weeks ago, he was completely unable to have an erection.

When you see Mark alone, he says he needs help "telling Susan about my 'real' problem." He states, "I've felt more and more uncomfortable with being a guy over the last 8 or 9 years. Even as a little kid, I played with dolls, and my mom sometimes dressed me in girls' clothes." Mark had male and female friends during his teens, but he was quite shy "so nobody seemed to care that I didn't date." When his friends began getting married, however, he started feeling social pressure to do so as well, and this bothered him. "I just tried to ignore my feelings at first, and when I met Susan 7 years ago, I thought things might be okay. She was a good friend." Mark married Susan, hoping that his ambivalent feelings "about being a guy" would subside over time. He valued her friendship and also initially enjoyed being sexually intimate with her. Over time, however, he found sexual contact to be less and less pleasurable. He reports, "During this past year, I have actually started wishing to be a real woman. I feel more and more like I should've been born female." He explains, "I didn't want to hurt Susan, so I would fake it, which worked all right for a while. I was afraid to tell her, because I feared she would feel betrayed. I found myself closing down instead, as she said. That's not like me."

Mark became increasingly unable to feel sexually aroused with his wife; maintaining an erection became impossible. However, he adds, "That's okay because I'm tired of this." When you ask for clarification, he explains, "I'm tired of being a man, not tired of sex. I have plenty of sexual desires, but I'll need to become a woman to fulfill them. Now I know that I want a sex change operation. Still, I don't want to hurt Susan, but I can't shut her out anymore either."

Clinical Presentation

Mark presents as a slim, well-dressed, groomed man who is alert and coherent. In the interview, he sits close to Susan and holds her hand, but he has infrequent eye contact and speaks little. Susan is also well dressed and groomed. She seems distressed and concerned but supportive toward Mark.

Once alone with you, Mark is no longer reserved and speaks freely. He appears generally calm but expresses frustration regarding his dilemma. When asked about his mood and state of mind in general, he replies, "pretty good, actually. This predicament is the only thing that pulls me down. I like my job, and frankly, I don't think having surgery would jeopardize my position. I have good friends, and I think the closest ones would understand. But I know I should tell Susan first, and I'm not sure how to do it."

Assessment Assumptions

All factors not explicitly mentioned above have been ruled out.

> **DSM-IV Axis I diagnosis:** 302.85 Gender identity disorder
> **DSM-IV Axis II diagnosis:** None

Identify the impairments on the next page.

Rating Impairment Severity   **41**

Step 1: Identifying Impairments

Instructions: *List **all the impairments, with behavioral evidence (statements/actions),** that accurately reflect Mark's current functioning on the Impairment Inventory below. List the impairments that refer **only to Mark**. Remember that information **not** mentioned should be assumed to be **nonapplicable** to this patient (e.g., no organic pathology is present). Assume that all symptoms and relevant information are reported in the case description.*

Impairment Inventory
1.
Behavioral evidence:
2.
Behavioral evidence:
3.
Behavioral evidence:
4.
Behavioral evidence:
5.
Behavioral evidence:

Turn the page for Impairment Inventory answers.

Impairment Inventory
(Impairments are listed chronologically as they appear in the vignette.)

1. Sexual Performance Dysfunction

Behavioral evidence: Mark has had increasing problems with maintaining an erection, culminating in complete failure during the last two attempts. He also doesn't want sex right now.

2. Uncommunicativeness

Behavioral evidence: After the first 3 years of marriage, Mark began sharing less about his feelings, often replying "I don't know" to Susan. Lately, he "hardly talks," is "closing down," and is "shutting her out."

3. Marital Dysfunction

Behavioral evidence: Mark has been "faking it" with Susan and has been "shutting her out" regarding his sexual identity concerns. Both Mark and Susan are dissatisfied with their sexual relationship but for different reasons. Role confusion will likely increase if/when Mark discloses.

4. Gender Dysphoria

Behavioral evidence: Mark has felt more and more uncomfortable with "being a guy" over the last 8 or 9 years. He has thoughts that he "should've been born female." During the past year, he has begun "wishing to be a real woman" and now is willing to have a sex change operation to accomplish this.

Common Errors

Anxiety: Mark does show "a state of uneasiness," but it is *not* "without sufficient objective justification." Rather, his concern over telling his wife of his Gender Dysphoria appears to be a legitimate cause of uneasiness.

Dysphoric Mood: This impairment describes general dysphoria, and Mark feels "pretty good, actually," with the exception of his Gender Dysphoria.

Rating Impairment Severity 43

Step 2: Rating Impairment Severity

Instructions: *Now provide severity ratings that accurately reflect Mark's current functioning, with rationales for each severity rating. Remember that the severity rationales requested below* **may overlap or be identical to** *the previously cited behavioral evidence for impairments. Information not mentioned should be assumed to be nonapplicable to this patient. Assume that all symptoms and relevant information are reported in the case description.*

Impairment Inventory	
Impairment	**Severity rating**
1. Sexual Performance Dysfunction	
Severity rationale:	
2. Uncommunicativeness	
Severity rationale:	
3. Marital Dysfunction	
Severity rationale:	
4. Gender Dysphoria	
Severity rationale:	

Turn the page for severity rating answers.

Impairment Inventory	
Impairment	**Severity rating**
1. Sexual Performance Dysfunction *(noncritical)*	**2** *(Destabilizing)*
Severity rationale: Mark has had increasing problems with maintaining an erection, culminating in complete failure during the last two attempts. He also doesn't want sex right now.	
2. Uncommunicativeness *(noncritical)*	**1** *(Distressing)*
Severity rationale: After the first 3 years of marriage, Mark began sharing less about his feelings, often replying "I don't know" to Susan. Lately, he "hardly talks," is "closing down," and is "shutting her out."	
3. Marital Dysfunction *(noncritical)*	**2** *(Destabilizing)*
Severity rationale: Mark has been "faking it" with Susan and has been "shutting her out" regarding his sexual identity concerns. Both Mark and Susan are dissatisfied with their sexual relationship but for different reasons. Role confusion will likely increase if/when Mark discloses.	
4. Gender Dysphoria *(noncritical)*	**2** *(Destabilizing)*
Severity rationale: Mark has felt more and more uncomfortable with "being a guy" over the last 8 or 9 years. He has thoughts that he "should've been born female." During the past year, he has begun "wishing to be a real woman" and now is willing to have a sex change operation to accomplish this.	

Common Errors

Gender Dysphoria: Given that Mark is very upset specifically about this impairment, a severity rating higher than 2 might seem appropriate. Note, however, that this is not a critical impairment, because it can never be "potentially/probably dangerous to oneself or others" nor can it "severely compromise self-care functioning." Remember that severities rate the extent to which an impairment causes *actual patient dysfunction;* they do *not* simply rate how upset the patient is about the impairment.

Sexual Performance Dysfunction: Similarly, Mark's "complete failure" in maintaining an erection might tempt some clinicians to rate this impairment severity as 4. This is inappropriate because Sexual Performance Dysfunction is not a critical impairment. Furthermore, Mark's functioning is "completely compromised" only regarding his attempts at maintaining an erection and not regarding his global self-care functioning. Remember that—for any noncritical impairment—*even complete dysfunction is denoted by a maximum severity of 2*, because noncritical impairments by definition cannot involve severe incapacitation or imminent danger.

Rating Impairment Severity

Notes

Turn the page for the next case.

Case Presentation 7
"Tamara"

Reason for Referral

Tamara, a 21-year-old African American woman, was referred to you for treatment after being treated in an emergency room for several cigarette burns on her arms. This was her fourth emergency room visit for this problem since age 17. This time, she was brought to the hospital by a neighbor who saw Tamara burning herself with a cigarette outside the apartment complex where they live. The neighbor noted that Tamara seemed "almost casual, like it didn't hurt!" Tamara initially refused the neighbor's offer for help and repeatedly stated, "Quit calling me Tamara, or I'll burn some more! My name is Angel." When her neighbor finally began calling Tamara "Angel," she then agreed to go to the emergency room. By the time she was seen by the physician, however, she once again answered to "Tamara." Furthermore, she did not remember calling herself "Angel," nor did she remember how her arms had gotten burned. You interview Tamara and her neighbor at the hospital and obtain the following information:

History

Tamara has been seen by various mental health professionals "since I was 10," and she has been treated at this hospital for cigarette burns three other times since age 17. Hospital records show that on two of these occasions, Tamara presented with marked agitation and insisted on calling herself "Angel"; on one occasion, she stated that "burns are good, and pain makes me stronger!" Records for all three incidents also show that several hours after being treated, Tamara was unable to recall how she was burned. Furthermore, she never remembered calling herself "Angel," nor did she know anyone by that name. Aside from these burn incidents, Tamara has no other history of self-injurious behavior.

After her last emergency room visit (6 months ago), she was transferred to a psychiatric inpatient facility where she remained under observation for 1 week and received no medication. Subsequently, Tamara began individual outpatient psychotherapy, but she stopped going after several sessions because "I didn't like the doctor."

Tamara attends a community college near her apartment, and she works at the college library to pay for expenses. She has dated sporadically but is not currently doing so. She reports having "only a few friends, probably because I'm so moody." When questioned about this, she explains, "People say I am way up one minute and way down the next. It's all the same to me, but everybody says it and I guess they can't all be wrong."

Clinical Presentation

Tamara presents as a slightly disheveled woman of average height and weight who is alert, coherent, and oriented. Her affect is unstable (i.e., rapidly fluctuating between tearful sadness and extremely cheerful laughter, etc.). When you ask her to describe her current feelings, she says, "I don't know. I've never been good at that. Happy, sad, it all seems pretty much the same. It's hard to describe, you know? Almost like I don't feel anything." Immediate, recent, and remote memory are all intact (with the exception of not remembering the burn incidents). Tamara views her neighbor as trustworthy and accepts the neighbor's claim that the current burns were self-inflicted. Still, she complains, "How can I stop doing something I don't remember? It's like there are these blank spots." Finally, when you ask her for her thoughts about "Angel," she becomes visibly more distressed and replies, "I wish people would believe me! I don't know anybody named Angel! Anyone who thinks I do know anybody by that name must be sicker than I am!"

Assessment Assumptions

No hallucinations or delusions are present, and there is no substance abuse. All factors not explicitly mentioned above have been ruled out.

> **DSM-IV Axis I diagnosis:** 300.14 Dissociative identity disorder
> **DSM-IV Axis II diagnosis:** None

Identify the impairments on the next page.

Rating Impairment Severity   47

Step 1: Identifying Impairments

Instructions: *List **all the impairments, with behavioral evidence (statements/actions),** that accurately reflect Tamara's current functioning on the Impairment Inventory below. List the impairments that refer **only to Tamara**. Remember that information **not** mentioned should be assumed to be **nonapplicable** to this patient (e.g., no organic pathology is present). Assume that all symptoms and relevant information are reported in the case description.*

Impairment Inventory
1.
Behavioral evidence:
2.
Behavioral evidence:
3.
Behavioral evidence:
4.
Behavioral evidence:
5.
Behavioral evidence:

Turn the page for Impairment Inventory answers.

Impairment Inventory
(Impairments are listed chronologically as they appear in the vignette.)

1. Self-Mutilation

Behavioral evidence: Tamara self-inflicted several cigarette burns on her arms. This is her fourth visit since age 17, with the last episode occurring 6 months ago. Otherwise, she has no history of self-injury.

2. Dissociative States

Behavioral evidence: She stated, "Quit calling me Tamara, or I'll burn some more! My name is Angel." Later, she did not remember calling herself "Angel," knows no one by that name, and did not remember how her arms were burned. This has been documented three times in 4 years.

3. Alexithymia

Behavioral evidence: When asked to describe her current feelings, she responds, "I don't know. I've never been good at that. Happy, sad, it all seems pretty much the same. It's hard to describe, you know? Almost like I don't feel anything."

4. Mood Lability

Behavioral evidence: Her affect is unstable, repeatedly shifting during the session (e.g., tearful sadness, extremely cheerful laughter).

Common Errors

Delusions (Nonparanoid):   Tamara's insistence that her name is "Angel" is clearly a belief that is "obviously contrary to demonstrable fact." This insistence has occurred on only three discrete occasions, however, and Tamara is unable to recall these events. Thus, calling herself "Angel" is limited to "disturbances or alterations in the normally integrative functions of identity, memory, or consciousness."

Dysphoric Mood: Although Tamara does show some moments of "apparent psychic suffering" (e.g., tearful sadness), this must be placed in the context of her *overall* mood, which is "unstable (i.e., rapidly fluctuating between tearful sadness and extremely cheerful laughter, etc.)." In addition, given her Alexithymia, her ability to communicate her own psychic suffering to a clinician is presumably impaired. Remember that identification of Dysphoric Mood requires behavioral evidence. Neither Tamara's actions (e.g., extremely cheerful laughter) nor her statements (e.g., "Almost like I don't feel anything") support the presence of Dysphoric Mood.

Rating Impairment Severity   **49**

Step 2: Rating Impairment Severity

Instructions: *Now provide severity ratings that accurately reflect Tamara's current functioning, with rationales for each severity rating. Remember that the severity rationales requested below* ***may overlap or be identical to*** *the previously cited behavioral evidence for impairments. Information not mentioned should be assumed to be nonapplicable to this patient. Assume that all symptoms and relevant information are reported in the case description.*

Impairment Inventory	
Impairment	**Severity rating**
1. Self-Mutilation	
Severity rationale:	
2. Dissociative States	
Severity rationale:	
3. Alexithymia	
Severity rationale:	
4. Mood Lability	
Severity rationale:	

Turn the page for the severity rating answers.

Impairment Inventory	
Impairment	**Severity rating**
1. Self-Mutilation *(critical)*	**2** *(Destabilizing)*
Severity rationale: Tamara self-inflicted several cigarette burns on her arms. This is her fourth visit since age 17, with the last episode occurring 6 months ago. Otherwise, she has no history of self-injury.	
2. Dissociative States *(critical)*	**2** *(Destabilizing)*
Severity rationale: She stated, "Quit calling me Tamara, or I'll burn some more! My name is Angel." Later, she did not remember calling herself "Angel," knows no one by that name, and she did not remember how her arms were burned. This has been documented three times in 4 years.	
3. Alexithymia *(noncritical)*	**2** *(Destabilizing)*
Severity rationale: When asked to describe her current feelings, she responds, "I don't know. I've never been good at that. Happy, sad, it all seems pretty much the same. It's hard to describe, you know? Almost like I don't feel anything."	
4. Mood Lability *(critical)*	**2** *(Destabilizing)*
Severity rationale: Her affect is unstable, repeatedly shifting during the session (e.g., tearful sadness, extremely cheerful laughter).	

Common Errors

Dissociative States: Some clinicians may want to assign a severity rating higher than 2 here, given that dissociative identity disorder is typically viewed as a serious diagnosis. Only three dissociative states have been documented in 4 years, however, and none of them has resulted in any severely incapacitating impairment. Note that *impairment severity is not determined by the type of diagnosis.* If additional incidents are documented and/or future incidents involve more extreme dysfunction, then this rating could increase to a 3 or 4.

Self-Mutilation: This impairment also is typically viewed as a severe type of dysfunction, prompting some clinicians to assign higher severity ratings. Tamara's behavior has been documented only four times in 4 years, however, and has never involved serious danger to self or others. Note that *impairment severity is not determined by the type of dysfunction (e.g., common, bizarre, rare) but by the degree of the resulting impairment.*

Notes

Turn the page for the next case.

52   **Casebook for Managing Managed Care**

Case Presentation 8

"Juan"

Reason for Referral

Juan, a 7-year-old Latino boy, was referred to you by Child Protective Services. Seven weeks ago, Juan reportedly began exhibiting some behaviors of concern at school. His teacher noticed one particular incident in which Juan and some other children were "playing house" during recess. Juan said that he was the "baby-sitter" and insisted that the other children "play doctor just like at my house when Mommy is gone." (Child Protective Services investigated the report made by his teacher, and Juan's 15-year-old baby-sitter, Tom, confessed to initiating mutual masturbation with Juan.) Since then, Juan's mother reports that Juan has been having trouble falling asleep, requesting that the hall light be left on (a new request), and is apparently having nightmares during which he awakens and screams out (e.g., "I don't want to!", "Tom!"). You see Juan and his mother and obtain the following information:

History

Juan lives alone with his mother (his father was killed in an automobile accident before Juan's first birthday). His mother works from 9:00 A.M. to 5:00 P.M. and was delighted to obtain Tom (recommended by a neighbor) as a baby-sitter to watch Juan after school. Juan has generally done average work in school, and school testing places him well within normal limits intellectually and academically. His teacher has noted, however, that he is very sensitive to criticism and has difficulty being accepted by his peers (although apparently he wants very much to be liked). Furthermore, when Juan approaches a new task, he becomes irritable and often says, "I'm stupid" or "I can't do this." When asked why he thinks so, he has told his teacher that "Tom says I am too dumb to do things myself. He must help me or I can't do things."

At home, Juan also has been somewhat temperamental lately. His mother reports that he has resisted her attempts to discuss Tom, but Juan does state emphatically, "Don't let him come over anymore, Mommy!" Since the incident with Tom, Juan has also shown markedly less affection. Formerly, he often instigated hugs and kisses, but now he does so only at his mother's request.

Clinical Presentation

You first see Juan's mother, who appears tense, occasionally angry, and generally distressed. She seems genuinely concerned for her son, and she interacts very well with him when Juan joins the two of you. On entering your office and having his mother introduce him, Juan heads straight for your sand tray and begins playing. He is neatly groomed and dressed in play clothes. Upon first meeting you, he is polite, calm, and does not appear shy, even when his mother leaves. During the session, however, he makes eye contact only occasionally; instead, he preferentially focuses on the toys in the sand tray. When you ask about his baby-sitter and his bad dreams, Juan stops talking, avoids all eye contact, and bangs the toys together. When you ask about the toys, however, he resumes speaking. When questioned about his schoolwork, he keeps playing and says, "I'm dumb. It's too hard."

Assessment Assumptions

All factors not explicitly mentioned above have been ruled out.

> **DSM-IV Axis I diagnosis:** 309.81 Posttraumatic stress disorder
> **DSM-IV Axis II diagnosis:** None

Identify the impairments on the next page.

Rating Impairment Severity   53

Step 1: Identifying Impairments

Instructions: *List **all the impairments, with behavioral evidence (statements/actions),** that accurately reflect Juan's current functioning on the Impairment Inventory below. List the impairments that refer **only to Juan**. Remember that information **not** mentioned should be assumed to be **nonapplicable** to this patient (e.g., no organic pathology is present). Assume that all symptoms and relevant information are reported in the case description.*

Impairment Inventory
1.
Behavioral evidence:
2.
Behavioral evidence:
3.
Behavioral evidence:
4.
Behavioral evidence:
5.
Behavioral evidence:

Turn the page for Impairment Inventory answers.

Impairment Inventory
(Impairments are listed chronologically as they appear in the vignette.)

1. Self-Esteem Deficiency

Behavioral evidence: Juan is very sensitive to criticism and has difficulty being accepted by peers. He says, "I'm stupid," "I can't do this," or "I'm dumb. It's too hard."

2. Emotional Abuse Victim

Behavioral evidence: Juan reports that "Tom says I am too dumb to do things myself. He must help me or I can't do things." These statements have contributed to a self-esteem deficiency and hinder Juan's optimal school performance.

3. Altered Sleep

Behavioral evidence: Juan has been having trouble falling asleep, requests that the hall light be left on (a new request), and apparently has nightmares during which he awakens and cries out (e.g., "I don't want to!", "Tom!").

4. Sexual Trauma Victim

Behavioral evidence: Juan's 15-year-old baby-sitter, Tom, confessed to mutual masturbation with Juan.

Common Errors

Anxiety: Juan does show "a state of uneasiness," but it is *not* "without sufficient objective justification." Rather, his fear of his baby-sitter appears to be the legitimate result of being a Sexual Trauma Victim.

Uncommunicativeness: Juan does appear to have some "unwillingness or inability to impart information, thoughts, or feelings to others." Specifically, when questioned about his baby-sitter and nightmares, "Juan stops talking, avoids all eye contact, and bangs the toys together." Note, however, that this behavior is documented only in the therapy setting, with the clinician, regarding only specific information. Otherwise, Juan communicates readily with all relevant parties (e.g., his mother, the clinician, teachers, peers). *To document an impairment, it is essential to show that the relevant behavior is not purely coincidental.* In this case, for example, Juan's resistance to talking about his sexual trauma might simply relate to hesitancy in self-disclosing potentially shame-provoking information to a stranger (the clinician). As such, Juan's behavior might relate to insufficient rapport between himself and the clinician.

Rating Impairment Severity 55

Step 2: Rating Impairment Severity

Instructions: *Now provide severity ratings that accurately reflect Juan's current functioning, with rationales for each severity rating. Remember that the severity rationales requested below* ***may overlap or be identical to*** *the previously cited behavioral evidence for impairments. Information not mentioned should be assumed to be nonapplicable to this patient. Assume that all symptoms and relevant information are reported in the case description.*

Impairment Inventory	
Impairment	**Severity rating**
1. Self-Esteem Deficiency	
Severity rationale:	
2. Emotional Abuse Victim	
Severity rationale:	
3. Altered Sleep	
Severity rationale:	
4. Sexual Trauma Victim	
Severity rationale:	

Turn the page for the severity rating answers.

Impairment Inventory	
Impairment	**Severity rating**
1. Self-Esteem Deficiency *(noncritical)*	**2** *(Destabilizing)*
Severity rationale: He is very sensitive to criticism and has difficulty being accepted by peers. He says, "I'm stupid," "I can't do this," or "I'm dumb. It's too hard."	
2. Emotional Abuse Victim *(noncritical)*	**1** *(Distressing)*
Severity rationale: Juan reports that "Tom says I am too dumb to do things myself. He must help me or I can't do things." These statements have contributed to a self-esteem deficiency and hinder Juan's optimal school performance.	
3. Altered Sleep *(noncritical)*	**1** *(Distressing)*
Severity rationale: He has been having trouble falling asleep, requests that the hall light be left on (a new request), and apparently has nightmares during which he awakens and cries out (e.g., "I don't want to!", "Tom!").	
4. Sexual Trauma Victim *(noncritical)*	**2** *(Destabilizing)*
Severity rationale: Juan's 15-year-old baby-sitter, Tom, confessed to mutual masturbation with Juan.	

Common Errors

Self-Esteem Deficiency: Because Juan's problem predates his sexual trauma and appears to be more long-standing, it might seem appropriate to assign a severity of 3. Severity ratings reflect the *current* level of impairment, however. Note that *they do not convey any information about the chronicity of a problem or its potential for repair.* An impairment with a severity of 4 might be rapidly and readily repairable, whereas an impairment with a severity of 1 might be long-standing and highly resistant to intervention.

Sexual Trauma Victim: Severity ratings higher than 2 are incorrect because this impairment is not critical. In order for a Sexual Trauma Victim to be severely incapacitated or in imminent danger, he or she *also* must have a critical impairment (e.g., Physical Abuse Victim). Note that *the same event might result in both noncritical and critical impairments.*

Rating Impairment Severity

Notes

Turn the page for the next case.

Case Presentation 9

"Wanda"

Reason for Referral

The R. family has been referred to you by the local high school counselor. Wanda R., a 14-year-old African American girl, has left school early (missing afternoon classes) and gone to a local park five times during the past 3 weeks. Wanda's maternal grandmother died a month ago, and Wanda has "been quite upset" since returning from the funeral. Although the school notified Mr. and Mrs. R. about these absences, they did not respond, and the situation has not changed. Because of these absences and because her teachers have noted that she looks "very sad," her school counselor recommended that Wanda and her parents meet with you. You interview the family and obtain the following information:

History

Mr. R. is a 43-year-old businessman, Mrs. R. is a 39-year-old real estate agent, and Wanda is an only child. As the session begins, you learn that Wanda's grandmother had lived 2,000 miles away, Wanda had spent time with her only on a handful of occasions, and Wanda did not really know her very well. Wanda remains quiet initially when asked about her school absences. With encouragement from her mother, however, she complies. Becoming tearful, she explains that she leaves school early to "spend time thinking about my grandmother. I really miss her." She appears to believe that her actions are a reasonable response to her grandmother's death, and her mother agrees. Specifically, Mrs. R. states that "Wanda is a sensitive child, and she's a real comfort to me. Everybody needs some time when they lose somebody close." Wanda also tells you that she leaves school early because she is "too tired to keep my mind on schoolwork—especially after lunch."

You ask her parents if they have noticed any significant changes in Wanda's behavior recently, to which Mrs. R. replies, "Not really. She hasn't had much of an appetite lately, but then neither have I. The school did call us about her cutting afternoon classes, but we didn't think there was anything to get too concerned about. Besides, she gets good grades, and one of the classes is just a study hall. I'm sure she'll get back on top of things in a week or two."

Clinical Presentation

Wanda presents as a quiet adolescent of age-appropriate height and weight. She is alert, coherent, and shows no evidence of hallucinations or delusions. She is somewhat sullen and appears to be holding back tears through much of the session. When she does speak, she includes a reference to her grandmother in almost every statement. When you ask Wanda what activities she enjoys, she replies, "nothing really lately. I just spend a lot of time hanging out and thinking about my Grandma. Besides, I'm tired all the time."

Wanda's father looks concerned and is generally quiet; however, he often sighs after his wife's comments. When you ask for his opinion, he hesitatingly replies, "I'm not sure about all this. To be completely honest, I think Wanda is taking this a bit too hard." Wanda's mother appears to be forcing a cheerful demeanor. She often looks at her husband when speaking for the both of them—as if to gain his support. The one time she becomes tearful, she bites her lip, and her husband changes the subject by talking about how Wanda helps out at home.

Assessment Assumptions

Wanda is not experiencing any abuse (i.e., substance, emotional, physical, sexual). All factors not explicitly mentioned above have been ruled out. While in your waiting room, Wanda completed the Children's Depression Inventory (Kovacs 1979). Her score was 2 standard deviations above the mean, suggesting significant symptomatology.

> **DSM-IV Axis I diagnosis:** 296.22 Major depression, single episode, moderate
> **DSM-IV Axis II diagnosis:** None

Identify the impairments on the next page.

Rating Impairment Severity   59

Step 1: Identifying Impairments

Instructions: *List **all the impairments, with behavioral evidence (statements/actions),** that accurately reflect Wanda's current functioning on the Impairment Inventory below. List the impairments that refer **only to Wanda**. Remember that information **not** mentioned should be assumed to be **nonapplicable** to this patient (e.g., there is no organic pathology). Assume that all symptoms and/or relevant information are reported in the case description.*

Impairment Inventory
1.
Behavioral evidence:
2.
Behavioral evidence:
3.
Behavioral evidence:
4.
Behavioral evidence:
5.
Behavioral evidence:

Turn the page for Impairment Inventory answers.

Impairment Inventory

(Impairments are listed chronologically as they appear in the vignette.)

1. Truancy

Behavioral evidence: Wanda has left school (missing afternoon classes) and gone to a local park five times during the past 3 weeks.

2. Pathological Grief

Behavioral evidence: Wanda reportedly skips classes to think about her grandmother, even though she seldom saw her and did not know her well. She also spends much time "just hanging out and thinking about my Grandma." She seems to include a reference to her grandmother in almost every statement.

3. Dysphoric Mood

Behavioral evidence: Wanda's teachers have noticed that she looks "very sad" in class. She is sullen and apparently holding back tears through much of the session. Regarding activities she enjoys, she states, "nothing really lately." Her score on the Children's Depression Inventory was 2 standard deviations above the mean, suggesting a significant symptomatology.

4. Family Dysfunction

Behavioral evidence: Wanda's parents did nothing about her absences, even when notified. Her mother thinks that Wanda's pathological grief is a reasonable response. Her parents "didn't think there was anything to get too concerned about." Her mother generally speaks for both parents, and her father only hesitatingly replies, even when questioned directly. When her mother's forced cheerfulness is once broken by tears, she bites her lip, and her husband changes the subject.

Common Errors

Decreased Concentration: Wanda does state that she is "too tired to keep my mind on schoolwork—especially after lunch." This does not clearly reflect a "reduction in *ability* to direct one's thoughts or efforts to sustain attention," however. The overall clinical picture suggests that Wanda's reported difficulties with schoolwork after lunch are *motivational* and reflect a rationalization for her tardiness. Also, her teachers cite no concentration problems. Note that *an impairment is not documented merely because a patient states its presence. Rather, statements (and actions) provide support for the clinician's conclusion that an impairment is present.*

School Avoidance: Wanda has shown several instances of "refusal to attend school," but this has only involved afternoons, and she has attended school even on these days. Furthermore, her absences have not been in order to "stay with major attachment figures."

Step 2: Rating Impairment Severity

Instructions: *Now provide severity ratings that accurately reflect Wanda's current functioning, with rationales for each severity rating. Remember that the severity rationales requested below **may overlap or be identical to** the previously cited behavioral evidence for impairments. Information not mentioned should be assumed to be nonapplicable to this patient. Assume that all symptoms and relevant information are reported in the case description.*

Impairment Inventory	
Impairment	**Severity rating**
1. Truancy	
Severity rationale:	
2. Pathological Grief	
Severity rationale:	
3. Dysphoric Mood	
Severity rationale:	
4. Family Dysfunction	
Severity rationale:	

Turn the page for the severity rating answers.

Impairment Inventory	
Impairment	**Severity rating**
1. Truancy *(noncritical)*	**1** *(Distressing)*
Severity rationale: Wanda has left school (missing afternoon classes) and gone to a local park five times during the past 3 weeks. Her grades in school are still good.	
2. Pathological Grief *(noncritical)*	**2** *(Destabilizing)*
Severity rationale: Wanda skips classes to think about her grandmother, even though she seldom saw her and did not know her well. In addition, she spends much time "just hanging out and thinking about my Grandma." She seems to include a reference to her grandmother in almost every statement.	
3. Dysphoric Mood *(critical)*	**2** *(Destabilizing)*
Severity rationale: Wanda's teachers have noticed that she looks "very sad" in class. She is sullen and apparently holding back tears through much of the session. Regarding activities she enjoys, she states, "nothing really lately." Her score on the Children's Depression Inventory was 2 standard deviations above the mean, suggesting a significant symptomatology.	
4. Family Dysfunction *(noncritical)*	**2** *(Destabilizing)*
Severity rationale: Wanda's parents did nothing about her absences, even when notified. Her mother thinks that Wanda's pathological grief is a reasonable response. Her parents "didn't think there was anything to get too concerned about." Her mother generally speaks for both parents, and her father only hesitatingly replies, even when questioned directly. When her mother's forced cheerfulness is once broken by tears, she bites her lip, and her husband changes the subject.	

Common Error

Pathological Grief: This impairment also might be viewed as a severe type of dysfunction, given that it is less common than other impairments. Pathological Grief is not a critical impairment, however, and can receive only a maximum severity of 2. More severe dysfunction, if present, would be attributed to Wanda's Dysphoric Mood, which is a more general impairment. Note that *impairment severity is not determined by dysfunction type (e.g., uncommon, bizarre, common), but rather by the degree of resulting impairment.*

Notes

Turn the page for the next case.

64   Casebook for Managing Managed Care

Case Presentation 10
"Carlos"

Reason for Referral

Carlos, a 41-year-old Latino man, was referred to you for evaluation by the county prison. You evaluate him there, where you occasionally provide consultations. Carlos is charged with arson and attempted murder. He is handcuffed when escorted to the evaluation room by an officer who then waits just outside the door. Carlos was arrested after setting fire to his former girlfriend's mobile home 2 nights ago while she was asleep inside. She lost her home but was unharmed. Carlos's public defender has requested a diagnostic evaluation. You interview Carlos and obtain the following information:

History

Carlos reports having seen "a lot of counselors" since elementary school "for fighting, skipping school, snagging pocketbooks, whatever." He "hate[s] counselors almost as much as cops, because they always butt their noses in and it never helps." Carlos boasts of a long adult criminal record, starting with arrests for stealing and vandalism, and, more recently, for drug sales and automobile theft. He also has been arrested for assault several times "when I was dumb enough to get caught. I've never been nabbed for my best fights." When questioned further, he explains, "if anybody gets in my face, I slam 'em. End of story!" He has been free on parole for the last 9 months, which is his longest interval between imprisonments as an adult.

   Carlos met his former girlfriend Linda, a 36-year-old Latina woman, shortly after leaving prison. They lived together for 6 months, but "she was always on my case and was getting too possessive." A week ago, one of Linda's friends told her she saw Carlos talking to another woman at a local bar. Carlos and Linda argued when she questioned him, and "she kicked me out! But nobody kicks me out and gets away with it, so I figured I'd teach her a lesson." When you ask him about the possible consequences of his actions, Carlos replies that "if she was too dumb to wake up when she smelled smoke, it would have served her right."

Clinical Presentation

Carlos presents as a tall, slightly overweight, acceptably groomed man. He is alert, coherent, and generally cooperative. His speech is normal but lacks full emotional expressiveness. He sneers often, rarely making eye contact. He appears calm and rarely shifts in his seat throughout the interview. When asked how he feels about his current situation, he smiles and says that "I am sorry I got caught, but being locked up doesn't bug me. I've sure lived in worse places than prison, and I can look out for myself okay." When asked how he feels about his recent actions, he replies, "I feel fine. Why?"

   Carlos reveals that he and Linda paid expenses by selling stolen merchandise but adds, "the cops could never prove that." He denies any substance abuse, explaining that "you can't sell and use at the same time," and laboratory tests support his denial. When asked about his feelings for Linda, he replies, "I'm glad it's all over between us." He also volunteers that her "kicking me out like dirt did make me angry." When asked about the fire, he states, "It's the first one I ever got caught for, but it was worth it!" When questioned further, he says, "I've always gotten a kick out of torching things! It helps me cool off, too!" When asked if he had intended to kill Linda, he again smiles and states, "if I really wanted to kill her, I guess she'd probably be dead, wouldn't she?"

Assessment Assumptions

No substance abuse is present. All factors not explicitly mentioned above have been ruled out.

> **DSM-IV Axis I diagnosis:** None
> **DSM-IV Axis II diagnosis:** 301.7 Antisocial personality disorder

Identify the impairments on the next page.

Rating Impairment Severity   65

Step 1: Identifying Impairments

Instructions: *List **all the impairments, with behavioral evidence (statements/actions),** that accurately reflect Carlos's current functioning on the Impairment Inventory below. List the impairments that refer **only to Carlos**. Remember that information **not** mentioned should be assumed to be **nonapplicable** to this patient (e.g., there is no organic pathology). Assume that all symptoms and/or relevant information are reported in the case description.*

Impairment Inventory
1.
Behavioral evidence:
2.
Behavioral evidence:
3.
Behavioral evidence:
4.
Behavioral evidence:
5.
Behavioral evidence:

Turn the page for Impairment Inventory answers.

Impairment Inventory
(Impairments are listed chronologically as they appear in the vignette.)

1. Fire Setting

Behavioral evidence: Carlos placed his former girlfriend in life-threatening danger by setting fire to her mobile home 2 nights ago while she slept inside. He also admits to a history of fire setting, stating that "I've always gotten a kick out of torching things! It helps me cool off, too!"

2. Stealing

Behavioral evidence: Carlos has a long history of theft beginning in his youth (e.g., he was reportedly apprehended for "snagging" pocketbooks). There are reports of recent stealing as well (e.g., automobile theft; Carlos and Linda paid their expenses by selling stolen merchandise).

3. Homicidal Thought/Behavior

Behavioral evidence: Carlos is currently held on attempted murder and arson charges. He also states that "if [his former girlfriend] was too dumb to wake up when she smelled smoke, it would have served her right."

4. Egocentricity

Behavioral evidence: He shows empathic failure regarding his former girlfriend by stating, "if she was too dumb to wake up when she smelled smoke, it would have served her right."

5. Assaultiveness

Behavioral evidence: He has been arrested for assault several times "when I was dumb enough to get caught. I've never been nabbed for my best fights." When questioned further, Carlos explains that "if anybody gets in my face, I slam 'em. End of story!"

Common Errors

Externalization and Blame: Carlos does state that "nobody kicks me out and gets away with it, so I figured I'd teach her a lesson." This statement does not actually involve blame, however. Rather, it merely reflects his acknowledgment of being angered by his former girlfriend's response to his behavior.

Marital/Relationship Dysfunction: Whereas the relationship between Carlos and Linda was clearly dysfunctional, Carlos now states, "I'm glad it's over between us." Note that *without a current relationship and/or desire for reconciliation, this impairment cannot logically be cited.*

Rating Impairment Severity 67

Step 2: Rating Impairment Severity

Instructions: *Now provide severity ratings that accurately reflect Carlos's current functioning, with rationales for each severity rating. Remember that the severity rationales requested below* **may overlap or be identical to** *the previously cited behavioral evidence for impairments. Information not mentioned should be assumed to be nonapplicable to this patient. Assume that all symptoms and relevant information are reported in the case description.*

Impairment Inventory	
Impairment	**Severity rating**
1. Fire Setting	
Severity rationale:	
2. Stealing	
Severity rationale:	
3. Homicidal Thought/Behavior	
Severity rationale:	
4. Egocentricity	
Severity rationale:	
5. Assaultiveness	
Severity rationale:	

Turn the page for the severity rating answers.

Impairment Inventory	
Impairment	**Severity rating**
1. Fire Setting *(critical)*	**4** *(Imminently dangerous)*
Severity rationale: Carlos has placed his former girlfriend in life-threatening danger by setting fire to her mobile home 2 nights ago while she slept inside. He also admits a history of fire setting.	
2. Stealing *(noncritical)*	**2** *(Destabilizing)*
Severity rationale: Carlos has a long history of theft (e.g., "snagging" pocketbooks as a youth) that extends to the present (e.g., automobile theft; Carlos and Linda paid their expenses by selling stolen merchandise).	
3. Homicidal Thought/Behavior *(critical)*	**4** *(Imminently dangerous)*
Severity rationale: Carlos is currently held on attempted murder and arson charges. He admits setting fire to his former girlfriend's trailer while she was inside asleep.	
4. Egocentricity *(noncritical)*	**2** *(Destabilizing)*
Severity rationale: He shows empathic failure regarding his former girlfriend by stating, "if she was too dumb to wake up when she smelled smoke, it would have served her right."	
5. Assaultiveness *(critical)*	**4** *(Imminently dangerous)*
Severity rationale: He has been arrested for assault several times "when I was dumb enough to get caught. I've never been nabbed for my best fights." He further states, "if anybody gets in my face, I slam 'em. End of story!"	

Common Error

Egocentricity: Some clinicians might wish to rate Carlos's Egocentricity as a 3 or even a 4 because of his extreme empathic failure regarding the life of his former girlfriend (i.e., "[I]f she was too dumb to wake up when she smelled smoke, it would have served her right."). However, this lack of empathy cannot directly result in severe incapacitation or imminent danger regarding self or others. Instead, Carlos's Egocentricity probably contributed to his decision to act on his homicidal thoughts. It was his Homicidal Thought/Behavior, however, that resulted in imminent danger. Note that *severe dysfunction signals the presence of a critical impairment.*

Rating Impairment Severity

The preceding five cases have illustrated how the clinician can begin patient assessments by taking an inventory of specific patient dysfunctions (i.e., impairments). As stated at the beginning of this chapter, an impairment's presence does *not* automatically indicate that it will be a focus of treatment.

First, to justify an impairment as a treatment focus, the clinician must be convinced that treatment is possible. Assessing treatment feasibility involves various factors. Does the patient perceive the dysfunction as a problem? Does the patient wish to repair the impairment? Does the patient have the psychological resources needed to engage in treatment of the impairment? Do research findings—if available—support the feasibility of treatment? Such questions will require answers before an identified impairment can be considered a focus of treatment. For example, in Case 10, no Patient Impairment Profile (PIP) could be constructed based on Carlos's Impairment Inventory. Specifically, none of his impairments causes him subjective distress, and he is not motivated to change in any way. When asked how he feels about his current situation, he smiles and says, "I am sorry I got caught, but being locked up doesn't bug me. I've sure lived in worse places than prison, and I can look out for myself okay." When asked how he feels about his recent actions, he replies, "I feel fine. Why?" This lack of distress and motivation to change is also consistent with his DSM-IV diagnosis (301.7 antisocial personality disorder). As such, Carlos's case exemplifies how the Impairment Inventory can be used to assess dysfunction, even when treatment is not indicated.

Second, to justify independent treatment for an impairment, the clinician must determine that it is not subsumed under another impairment. Specifically, clinical assessment may conclude that one impairment (e.g., Decreased Concentration) is entirely due to the presence of another (e.g., Pathological Grief). In such instances, the former impairment might not receive direct attention because it is expected to repair spontaneously with the treatment of the latter impairment.

Third, the clinician must determine the timing of treatment. Should a given impairment be treated now or at a later date? Although the severity of each impairment will inform these choices, the clinician's expertise will provide the ultimate basis for such timing decisions.

Assessing treatment feasibility, evaluating which identified impairments are independent treatment foci, and determining the appropriate timing of treatment for each impairment are three essential steps involved in the process of constructing a PIP based on an Impairment Inventory. Building the PIP is the subject of the next chapter.

The Patient Impairment Profile

This chapter explains the Patient Impairment Profile (PIP). Whereas an Impairment Inventory simply lists potential reasons for treatment, the PIP documents the clinician's prioritized decisions about what will actually be treated. As such, the PIP provides the basis for all communication between clinicians and reviewers. For the five new cases presented in this chapter, impairment identification and severity rating are combined into one step. Then, the clinician will use the resultant Impairment Inventories to create PIPs. For each case, answers with rationales follow each exercise, and common errors are also explained.

Definitions

level of care   The treatment setting; a type of unit, facility, or other location where a treatment approach or modality is offered.

Patient Impairment Profile (PIP)   The impairments that are prioritized as the focus of treatment and their respective severity ratings.

Chapter 3 illustrated the utility of taking a simple inventory of impairments, with their severities, for identifying potential reasons for treatment. As previously stated, however, the fact that a patient has a particular impairment does not automatically mandate the treatment of that impairment. For example, Case 10 (Carlos) showed how the Impairment Inventory could be used to assess a patient *for whom no treatment would be recommended.*

Once an Impairment Inventory is taken, the clinician must decide which *potential* reasons for treatment will become *actual* treatment foci. The clinician also must strengthen the clinical rationale for treatment by prioritizing the impairments to be treated. This task is simplified both by impairment severities and by impairment classification (i.e., as either critical or noncritical). First, impairments receiving higher severities logically merit priority. Thus, an impairment with a severity of 3 should be ranked higher in a PIP than one with a severity of 2. Second, critical impairments by their nature make them likely candidates for more intense service settings than noncritical impairments, particularly because they can, by definition, receive severities of either 3 or 4. Finally, the impairment with the highest severity in a PIP will logically inform decisions about the appropriate type of treatment. Treatment type, in turn, will influence what *level of care* is needed.

The clinician's judgment is the final decision-making standard for prioritizing impairments, however. First, a patient might manifest both a critical impairment (e.g., Psychotic Thought/Behavior) with a severity of 1 and a noncritical impairment (e.g., Tantrums) with a severity of 2. When this occurs, the clinician might be well advised to target the noncritical impairment as the top priority. Second, often a patient may have several impairments with identical severities. Again, the clinician's judgment is the ultimate basis for ranking treatment foci. Even in such cases, however, the critical versus noncritical impairment distinction—with the severity ratings—can facilitate decision making. Specifically, if two cited impairments have identical severities (e.g., both are rated 2) but only one is a critical impairment, then the critical one should typically receive priority in the PIP.

When developing a PIP, the clinician must remember that only those impairments *actually present currently* should be cited. This might initially be counterintuitive for clinicians accustomed to diagnosing "underlying" problems that are not currently manifest. For example, if a young patient has Tantrums, many clinicians might assume that she or he is also experiencing Family Dysfunction (e.g., poor parenting). However, this latter impairment would not be listed on the PIP unless supportive behavioral evidence (i.e., statements or actions) was found at the time of assessment. Instead, because the PIP is not a static document, it may be appropriate for a clinician to include "assess for Family Dysfunction" as a proposed intervention (see Chapter 6) for the Tantrums. Then, when updating the PIP later, the second impairment could be added if it was supported with behavioral evidence. This dynamic (versus static) approach to describing patient impairments also facilitates communication of a clinical rationale for continued treatment needs (e.g., when additional impairments do surface and are identified). In addition, identifying only *currently observable and behaviorally supportable* impairments prevents the clinician from "stuffing" the PIP and sharpens treatment focus, making treatment authorization more likely.

Step 3: Creating the Patient Impairment Profile

Five new cases follow, providing you the opportunity to integrate Step 1 (Identifying Impairments) and Step 2 (Rating Impairment Severity) into one step (Creating the Impairment Inventory). Thus, your behavioral evidence will combine support for each cited impairment with justification of each severity rating. After reviewing the Impairment Inventory answers and rationales for a case, you will

The Patient Impairment Profile **73**

use this information to construct its Patient Impairment Profile (PIP). As in Chapter 3, please read the vignette and imagine that you are actually interviewing the patient. Then complete the Impairment Inventories and PIPs, and compare them with the answers that follow.

74   Casebook for Managing Managed Care

Case Presentation 11

"April"

Reason for Referral

April, a 35-year-old Asian American woman, was referred to you by her independent living coordinator, who states, "I would've called April's psychiatrist, but she is on vacation and she gave me your number for emergencies." April has been acting bizarre recently and has shown generally poor judgment. Several days ago, her coordinator found April placing her pet cat in a pot on the stove with the heat turned on high. April's behavior changes have been apparent for about 2 weeks. You interview April with her coordinator and obtain the following information:

History

April never completed high school, and she is functionally illiterate. She reports no interest in learning to read, stating, "I prefer television." April has a history of mental and emotional problems (for which she has received medication) since age 18 years. After a series of hospitalizations, she was placed in a structured and supervised group home when she was 25. She did relatively well in this setting and 12 months ago "took a real turn for the better" according to her independent living coordinator. As a result, 9 months ago, she was moved to a semi-independent living situation (her own efficiency apartment on the group home grounds). She seemed to do well in this setting, demonstrating acceptable social skills and appropriate judgment. Given this progress and because she began to complain of some extrapyramidal side effects from her Haldol (haloperidol 20 mg/day), her medication was reduced to 15 mg/day and later to 10 mg/day.

According to her coordinator, April "took a turn for the worse about 2 weeks ago and started acting crazier than she has in years. We ruled out substance abuse, but it might be her medication because it was just reduced again." The coordinator further states that "lately, April's social skills have gone out the window, too. She often makes inappropriate comments and interrupts others during group therapy, and her constant cackling laughter is pushing us all to the limit!" For the past month, April also has shown increasingly poor judgment in general, and she has become "dangerously forgetful." Her coordinator has inferred April's forgetfulness from the fact that April has left electric appliances running on several occasions. Furthermore, her coordinator states that "April is acting so strangely that she must be watched constantly now."

Clinical Presentation

April is a slender woman who is casually dressed, demonstrates acceptable hygiene, and appears to be in good health. During the interview, her speech is often incoherent (e.g., "You must be a nice doctor because it isn't raining after all."), and her associations are very loose (e.g., "I don't have new clothes for the party, but I respect Libertarians."). She is oriented to person, time, and place and denies hallucinations. Her mood is positive, but her affect is flat or inappropriate. When asked why she put her cat on the stove, she laughs and says, "to heat the extra electricity out of her, of course! There are too many electrical currents in my apartment." You also discover that she does *not* "forget" to turn off her appliances (her memory is within normal limits). Rather, she intentionally leaves them running "to get rid of the extra electricity." When you ask her about her beliefs regarding electricity and suggest that she may have been experiencing some additional stress recently, she laughs again, stating, "That's silly. I feel real good. I like electricity when I take a nap."

Assessment Assumptions

All factors not explicitly mentioned above have been ruled out.

> **DSM-IV Axis I diagnosis**: 295.10 Schizophrenia, disorganized type
> **DSM-IV Axis II diagnosis**: None

Identify the impairments and rate their severities on the next page.

The Patient Impairment Profile   75

Steps 1 & 2:
Identifying Impairments and Rating Severity

Instructions: *List **all the impairments,** with their respective **severity ratings.** After each, cite **behavioral evidence (statements/actions)** that supports your choices of both impairments and severities. List the impairments that refer **only to April.** Remember that information **not** mentioned should be assumed to be **nonapplicable** to this patient (e.g., no organic pathology is present). Assume that all symptoms and/or relevant information are reported in the case description.*

Impairment Inventory	
Impairment	**Severity rating**
1.	
Behavioral evidence:	
2.	
Behavioral evidence:	
3.	
Behavioral evidence:	
4.	
Behavioral evidence:	
5.	
Behavioral evidence:	

Turn the page for Impairment Inventory and severity rating answers.

Impairment Inventory	
(Impairments are chronologically listed as they appear in the vignette.)	
Impairment	**Severity rating**
1. Educational Performance Deficit *(noncritical)*	**2** *(Destabilizing)*
Behavioral evidence: April never completed high school, and she is functionally illiterate; she reports no interest in learning to read, stating, "I prefer television." Her functional illiteracy (and current lack of motivation to become literate) markedly interferes with her ability to care for herself (e.g., preventing employment and completely independent living).	
2. Psychotic Thought/Behavior *(critical)*	**3** *(Severely incapacitating)*
Behavioral evidence: April engages in grossly disorganized, unexplainable behaviors (e.g., constant cackling laughter). She resists alternative explanations of her thoughts and behaviors and is markedly illogical (e.g., "That's silly. I feel real good. I like electricity when I take a nap.").	
3. Delusions (Nonparanoid) *(critical)*	**4** *(Imminently dangerous)*
Behavioral evidence: April has beliefs that are obviously contrary to demonstrable fact (e.g., putting her cat on the stove "to heat the extra electricity out of her, of course!" and leaving her appliances on to overheat and "get rid of the extra electricity"). She also acts on her delusions, putting herself and others in imminent danger. These frequently life-threatening behaviors require her to "be watched constantly now" according to her coordinator.	
4. Inadequate Self-Maintenance Skills *(noncritical)*	**2** *(Destabilizing)*
Behavioral evidence: April's coordinator states that April's "social skills have gone out the window. She often makes inappropriate comments, and she often interrupts others during group therapy." April also has shown increasingly poor judgment in general and must be watched constantly.	

Common Errors

Assaultiveness: April's actions do "potentially harm…animals," but they are not "acts of physical violence." Rather, she placed her cat on the stove because of her delusion that it would help to "heat the extra electricity out of her."

Learning Disability: April's illiteracy is functional and has a motivational component (e.g., "I prefer television."). Before concluding that she has a Learning Disability, formal assessment must be done. Thus, "assess for Learning Disability" could be cited as an intervention (see Chapter 6) for her Educational Performance Deficit.

Create the Patient Impairment Profile (PIP) on the next page.

The Patient Impairment Profile
77

Step 3: Creating the Patient Impairment Profile

Instructions: *Now, select those impairments from April's Impairment Inventory that will be the current focus of treatment. List them with their respective severity ratings on the Patient Impairment Profile below. List the impairments in **prioritized order.** Then, in the space below, write your rationale for your ranking of each. Remember that information **not** mentioned should be assumed to be **nonapplicable** to this patient.*

Patient Impairment Profile	
Impairment	**Severity rating**
1.	
2.	
3.	
4.	

1. Prioritization rationale:

2. Prioritization rationale:

3. Prioritization rationale:

4. Prioritization rationale:

Turn the page for prioritized PIP answers.

Case Presentation 11: April	
Patient Impairment Profile	
Impairment	**Severity rating**
1. Delusions (Nonparanoid)	4
2. Psychotic Thought/Behavior	3
3. Inadequate Self-Maintenance Skills	2
4. Educational Performance Deficit	2

1. Prioritization rationale: April's delusions must be addressed first because she is acting on them (e.g., leaving appliances running and putting her cat on the stove, creating an immediate fire hazard), and they are placing herself and others in imminent danger (severity of 4).

2. Prioritization rationale: April's Psychotic Thought/Behavior (e.g., marked illogicality and loose associations) must be addressed second because it is severely incapacitating (severity of 3) her ability to function (e.g., constant laughter).

3. Prioritization rationale: Attending to April's poor social skills and generally poor judgment could be considered the tertiary treatment focus. This impairment is destabilizing (severity of 2), particularly because it results in the disruption of her group therapy.

4. Prioritization rationale: April's functional illiteracy markedly inhibits her ability to pursue optimal levels of independent living. This destabilizing concern (severity of 2) may also merit increased attention as more severe impairments improve.

Common Error

Psychotic Thought/Behavior: Some clinicians might be tempted to place this impairment first in the PIP because April shows a wider *variety* of behaviors supporting its presence. Remember, however, that impairment prioritization is influenced by severities rather than simply by the number of statements/actions cited to support a given impairment. In this case, April's Delusions (severity of 4) are the primary treatment focus because they represent the greatest threat to her and others, even though she is having more Psychotic Thoughts/Behaviors than Delusions. Confusion can also result from the fact that the term *psychotic*—as generally used by mental health professionals—can be assumed to reflect a more severe level of global dysfunction than the term *delusion*. In fact, delusions can certainly be viewed as one type of psychotic thought. When using the Impairment Lexicon, however, the clinician must remember that *strict adherence to the operational definitions of terms is essential to ensure reliability*. Thus, on the Impairment Lexicon, Psychotic Thought/Behavior is "distinguished from Delusions" and vice versa. As such, Delusions are viewed as separate from Psychotic Thought/Behavior *for the purpose of communication via the PIP*.

The Patient Impairment Profile

Notes

Turn the page for the next case.

80   Casebook for Managing Managed Care

Case Presentation 12

"Billy"

Reason for Referral

Billy, a 5-year-old African American boy, was referred to you by friends of his parents. Billy has reportedly become increasingly "nervous" since he wet his bed 10 days ago during his first overnight stay outside the home (grandmother's home, 10 miles away). Since then, he has continuously apologized for "messing Grandma's bed" and states several times a day that he "didn't mean to do it." His parents are also distressed; they feel this represents a significant change in Billy's behavior. You interview Billy and his parents and obtain the following information:

History

Billy lives with his parents and is an only child. His parents describe his developmental milestones (e.g., toilet training) as normal and state that he does well in the accelerated kindergarten he attends. He has friends both in school and at home, and his teachers comment that he is cheerful, well behaved, and bright for his age. Billy's only problem has been a failure to develop full nocturnal bladder control; bed-wetting still occurs 2 or 3 nights per week. His parents, who have thus far simply been supportive of Billy, are now beginning to wonder if they might need to change their approach. His mother states, "Until recently, his accidents didn't seem to bother him in the least. Sure, he'd say he was sorry, but then he'd be fine as soon as we remade the bed together. We never scolded him because I guess we hoped he would just grow out of it."

Billy's father reports that they decided to let him stay overnight with his grandmother "so he knows we don't think he's still a baby." The visit was without incident except for Billy's bed-wetting. Billy's grandmother reported, however, that he had tried to make the bed so that she would not discover the accident. She came in the room before he finished, however, and Billy began repeatedly apologizing and saying, "Don't be mad." He also became distressed when she insisted on making the bed herself. Since Billy returned home, Billy's parents state that he frequently brings up the matter, repeatedly apologizing, despite his parents' continued assurances that no one is mad at him. His parents add that "over the last few days, he's started to seem nervous in general, not just about his accident."

Clinical Presentation

Billy presents as a neatly dressed and groomed boy of normal weight and height. He is well behaved and generally cheerful. Throughout the session, however, he appears tense and worried (e.g., hypervigilant, swings feet), particularly when his parents describe the bed-wetting incident. When asked, he says he knows that "Mommy and Daddy aren't mad." With further questioning, he reveals, "I don't know how to stop messing. I can't help it." He also fears that "Grandma won't let me visit anymore, and Mommy and Daddy will think I'm still a baby." Once during the session, he spontaneously apologizes to *you* for his "accident."

Billy's parents appear to get along and communicate well with each other during the interview. Their nurturing behavior toward Billy is appropriate. They wonder whether his grandmother (father's mother) might have reacted sternly.

Assessment Assumptions

No sexual or physical abuse is present. All factors not explicitly mentioned above have been ruled out.

> **DSM-IV Axis I diagnosis**: 307.6 Enuresis, nocturnal only
> **DSM-IV Axis II diagnosis:** None

Identify the impairments and rate their severities on the next page.

The Patient Impairment Profile   **81**

Steps 1 & 2:
Identifying Impairments and Rating Severity

Instructions: *List **all the impairments,** with their respective **severity ratings.** After each, cite **behavioral evidence (statements/actions)** that supports your choices of both impairments **and** severities. List the impairments that refer **only to Billy.** Remember that information **not** mentioned should be assumed to be **nonapplicable** to this patient (e.g., no organic pathology is present). Assume that all symptoms and/or relevant information are reported in the case description.*

Impairment Inventory	
Impairment	**Severity rating**
1.	
Behavioral evidence:	
2.	
Behavioral evidence:	
3.	
Behavioral evidence:	
4.	
Behavioral evidence:	
5.	
Behavioral evidence:	

Turn the page for Impairment Inventory and severity rating answers.

Impairment Inventory
(Impairments are listed chronologically as they appear in the vignette.)

Impairment	Severity rating
1. Enuresis *(noncritical)*	**1** *(Distressing)*
Behavioral evidence: Development (e.g., milestones, including toilet training) has been normal, and the only problem has been a failure to develop full nocturnal bladder control, with bed-wetting still occurring 2 or 3 nights per week.	
2. Pathological Guilt *(noncritical)*	**1** *(Distressing)*
Behavioral evidence: He has continued to apologize for "messing Grandma's bed" and has stated two or three times a day for the past 10 days that he "didn't mean to do it," despite his parents' continued assurances that no one is mad at him. He even spontaneously apologizes to *you* for his "accident."	
3. Anxiety *(critical)*	**1** *(Distressing)*
Behavioral evidence: His parents state that he has become increasingly "nervous in general, not just about his accident." In the session, he appears tense and worried (e.g., hypervigilant, swings feet). He states, "I don't know how to stop messing. I can't help it." He also fears that "Grandma won't let me visit anymore, and Mommy and Daddy will think I'm still a baby."	

Common Errors

Concomitant Medical Condition: Billy's bed-wetting is the typical form observed with nocturnal bladder control behavior. There is little reason to expect that it is due to medical problems. The responsible clinician will, however, ascertain whether appropriate physical examinations have been conducted. (This could be cited as an intervention for Enuresis: "Assess for Concomitant Medical Condition" [see Chapter 6].) If, in fact, a medical cause is found for his bed-wetting at a later date, then Concomitant Medical Condition would *replace* Enuresis in Billy's Impairment Inventory (see the Impairment Lexicon).

Dysphoric Mood: Billy is clearly distressed by his Enuresis, but this is manifested as anxiety and not Dysphoric Mood. In fact, Billy appears "well behaved and generally cheerful." Clinicians must avoid the tendency to confuse the specific Impairment Lexicon term *Dysphoric Mood* with more familiar terms (e.g., *upset, distressed,* and even *depressed*). Keep in mind that *strict adherence to the specific operational definitions in the Impairment Lexicon is necessary* for reliable communication (i.e., between clinicians and reviewers, etc.).

Create the Patient Impairment Profile (PIP) on the next page.

The Patient Impairment Profile   83

Step 3: Creating the Patient Impairment Profile

Instructions: *Now, select those impairments from Billy's Impairment Inventory that will be the current focus of treatment. List them with their respective severity ratings on the Patient Impairment Profile below. List the impairments in* **prioritized order.** *Then, in the space below, write your rationale for your ranking of each. Remember that information* **not** *mentioned should be assumed to be* **nonapplicable** *to this patient.*

Patient Impairment Profile	
Impairment	**Severity rating**
1.	
2.	
3.	

1. Prioritization rationale:

2. Prioritization rationale:

3. Prioritization rationale:

Turn the page for prioritized PIP answers.

Case Presentation 12: Billy	
Patient Impairment Profile	
Impairment	**Severity rating**
1. Enuresis	1
2. Pathological Guilt	1

1. Prioritization rationale: All of Billy's distressing (severity of 1) impairments seem to relate to Enuresis. Treatment options could include behavior therapy (e.g., moisture alarm) and/or medication. Enabling him to establish nocturnal bladder control will most likely result in the elimination of both Pathological Guilt and Anxiety.

2. Prioritization rationale: The clinician also should assess the degree to which Billy's guilt is merely a by-product of the events surrounding his first bed-wetting outside the home. If not, direct treatment of this impairment is appropriate. In either case, directly addressing the issue of guilt in play therapy might prove helpful. Anxiety seems closely tied to, and should resolve with successful treatment of, Pathological Guilt.

Common Error

Anxiety: Because this impairment is a critical one, some clinicians might automatically include it in the PIP and rank it as the top priority above the noncritical impairments. Keep in mind, however, that severity ratings take precedence over critical versus noncritical impairment classification when presenting a clinical rationale. In Billy's case, Anxiety was rated no higher than either Enuresis or Pathological Guilt (all three received a severity of 1), so its severity alone does not justify its being ranked first in the PIP.

As stated previously, if cited impairments have identical severities—but only one is a critical impairment—the critical one should *typically* receive priority in the PIP. This principle must never be seen as a decision *rule*, however, because exceptions occur. Billy's PIP presents one such exception that also clearly shows that the clinician's judgment is the ultimate basis for decisions. As the prioritization rationales above explain, Billy's Anxiety is most likely a by-product of the distress associated with his Pathological Guilt. If, in the future, Pathological Guilt resolves without a simultaneous remission of Anxiety, then this latter impairment could be included in the PIP at such time.

The Patient Impairment Profile

Notes

Turn the page for the next case.

86   **Casebook for Managing Managed Care**

Case Presentation 13

"Hannah"

Reason for Referral

Hannah, a 9-year-old Caucasian girl, and her parents were referred by Hannah's schoolteacher to you. Her teacher reportedly describes Hannah as "constantly restless and on the go." Her teacher is also concerned about Hannah's apparent difficulty with arithmetic and reading, leading to poor grades in these two areas. You interview Hannah and her mother (Hannah's father was not able to leave work for this meeting) and obtain the following information:

History

Hannah has an older brother (age 11) and a younger sister (age 6). Her parents have reportedly enjoyed a good marriage for 14 years. Hannah has never been to a "counselor" before, but her mother acknowledges that "she has always been very curious and fidgety, with more energy than both her brother and sister combined." Her mother adds, "She is also very distractible. In fact, she often doesn't even sit through her own favorite television shows." Hannah's mother also admits being concerned about an issue she describes as "somewhat of an embarrassment." Specifically, Hannah has never fully achieved sphincter control, and she still occasionally passes small amounts of stool in her clothes during the day. The family physician ruled out medical causes and suggested that Hannah might benefit from "psychological" help, but her parents "had really hoped we could solve this ourselves." "In fact," continues her mother, "she's down to about once a month now, and then it's usually on her way to the bathroom. It seems to happen when she's so active that she forgets or refuses to use the rest room, for fear that she'll miss something important." When you ask Hannah, she agrees, stating, "I don't like to miss any fun stuff." She also admits that she wants to stop soiling, however.

This year, Hannah switched from public to private school and is in fourth grade. She is reportedly described as an average student, but she apparently has difficulty staying in her seat during class. She also frequently fails to complete assigned tasks, leaving her seat or interrupting classmates instead. Her mother reports that public school teachers had made similar comments over the past 3 years, "but they thought she might grow out of it." Currently, Hannah also has difficulty getting along with her peers, often trying to join their games late or quitting shortly after beginning. She rarely waits her turn or plays quietly, and she talks excessively, often shouting out answers before questions are finished being read.

Recent testing (1 month ago) by the school psychologist indicates that Hannah's overall intellectual functioning is in the average range, with only one significant relative weakness. Specifically, her computational abilities are in the low average range. Her teacher says this is consistent with Hannah's "barely passing" arithmetic work in class.

Clinical Presentation

Hannah is a well-groomed and fully oriented girl of average height and weight. She is constantly fidgety, however, playing with her shoelaces, squirming in her chair, and often leaving her seat to walk around the room. She is cheerful and friendly and appears eager to please you, but she is also easily distracted and impulsive, often talking over you and answering your questions before you finish asking them. She states that she likes school, "except for math." When you question her further, she clarifies, "Math is too hard! I'd rather be in gym class." When asked about peer relationships, she responds, "I have lots of friends, but we don't get along so good sometimes."

Assessment Assumptions

All factors not explicitly mentioned above have been ruled out.

> **DSM-IV Axis I diagnosis:** 314.01 Attention-deficit/hyperactivity disorder
> **DSM-IV Axis I dual diagnosis:** 307.7 Encopresis
> **DSM-IV Axis I dual diagnosis:** 315.1 Mathematics disorder
> **DSM-IV Axis II diagnosis:** None

Identify the impairments and rate their severities on the next page.

The Patient Impairment Profile   87

Steps 1 & 2:
Identifying Impairments and Rating Severity

Instructions: *List **all the impairments,** with their respective **severity ratings.** After each, cite **behavioral evidence (statements/actions)** that supports your choices of both impairments and severities. List the impairments that refer **only to Hannah**. Remember that information **not** mentioned should be assumed to be **nonapplicable** to this patient (e.g., no organic pathology is present). Assume that all symptoms and/or relevant information are reported in the case description.*

Impairment Inventory	
Impairment	**Severity rating**
1.	
Behavioral evidence:	
2.	
Behavioral evidence:	
3.	
Behavioral evidence:	
4.	
Behavioral evidence:	
5.	
Behavioral evidence:	

Turn the page for Impairment Inventory and severity rating answers.

88   Casebook for Managing Managed Care

Impairment Inventory	
(Impairments are listed as they appear chronologically in the vignette.)	
Impairment	**Severity rating**
1. Motor Hyperactivity *(noncritical)*	**2** *(Destabilizing)*
Behavioral evidence: She is constantly restless and on the go, is fidgety, squirms in her chair, and often leaves her seat to walk around the room.	
2. Learning Disability *(noncritical)*	**1** *(Distressing)*
Behavioral evidence: Testing indicates that Hannah has a significant relative weakness in computational abilities (low average range), and she is "barely passing" arithmetic classwork. Hannah says, "Math is hard."	
3. Encopresis *(noncritical)*	**1** *(Distressing)*
Behavioral evidence: Hannah has never fully achieved sphincter control, and still occasionally (once monthly) passes small amounts of stool "on her way to the bathroom."	

Common Errors

Decreased Concentration: Although Hannah does have difficulty in "directing [her] thoughts or efforts to sustain attention," these problems reportedly have always been present. Thus, her concentration has not decreased and involves no "observed or reported reduction in ability."

Educational Performance Deficit: According to the Impairment Lexicon, an Educational Performance Deficit must be "not due to...learning disability." As such, the presence of Hannah's Learning Disability would make the citing of an Educational Performance Deficit not only incorrect but also redundant.

Create the Patient Impairment Profile (PIP) on the next page.

The Patient Impairment Profile

89

Step 3: Creating the Patient Impairment Profile

Instructions: *Now, select those impairments from Hannah's Impairment Inventory that will be the current focus of treatment. List them with their respective severity ratings on the Patient Impairment Profile below. List the impairments in **prioritized order.** Then, in the space below, write your rationale for your ranking of each. Remember that information **not** mentioned should be assumed to be **nonapplicable** to this patient.*

Patient Impairment Profile	
Impairment	**Severity rating**
1.	
2.	
3.	

1. Prioritization rationale:

2. Prioritization rationale:

3. Prioritization rationale:

Turn the page for prioritized PIP answers.

Case Presentation 13: Hannah	
Patient Impairment Profile	
Impairment	**Severity rating**
1. Motor Hyperactivity	2
2. Learning Disability	1
3. Encopresis	1

1. Prioritization rationale: Hannah's destabilizing activity levels (severity of 2) probably also exacerbate the effects of her learning disability and encopresis. Conversely, addressing her motor hyperactivity also might help to reduce her other two impairments. Treatment options might include medication and/or behavior therapy.

2. Prioritization rationale: If not addressed, this distressing (severity of 1) impairment is likely to have increasingly deleterious effects as Hannah continues her education. Treatment options might include referring Hannah for special education in math and therapeutically addressing emotional ramifications of this impairment.

3. Prioritization rationale: Because this impairment is not only distressing (severity of 1) but also long-standing, treatment is clearly indicated. Given the relatively circumscribed nature of this problem, complete eradication might be accomplished via a simple behavioral contract, including scheduled attempts to void (e.g., after meals).

Common Error

Encopresis: Because Encopresis is relatively less common than either a Learning Disability or Motor Hyperactivity in 9-year-old children, some clinicians might place this impairment first in the PIP. This impairment is compromising Hannah's overall functioning less than her other two impairments, however. As such, it is more appropriate to consider it as a simultaneous but tertiary focus of treatment. Remember that *neither impairment severity nor impairment prioritization in a PIP is influenced by the extent to which the problem is common versus unusual.*

The Patient Impairment Profile

Notes

Turn the page for the next case.

92   Casebook for Managing Managed Care

Case Presentation 14
"Zack"

Reason for Referral

Zack, a 30-year-old Caucasian man, has sought your services because his wife, Jean, a 31-year-old Caucasian woman, "insisted we get counseling if I wanted our marriage [of 4 years] to continue." After initially refusing to seek therapy, he finally agreed when he came home to find "she was actually packing." You see the couple, together and separately, and obtain the following information:

History

Zack works as a freelance musician "playing local gigs in bars and doing a lot of studio recording." Jean is a systems analyst for a large firm. They have a 3-year-old son, Zack Jr. Jean wanted "counseling" because of Zack's gambling—"he goes to the track all the time now, and he's always trying to win back his losses." Zack states that his "hobby is not worth fighting over. Besides, little bets aren't fun anymore, and it takes too long to win your money back." Jean states, however, that they are $9,000 in debt, and court-ordered garnishment of her paychecks has begun. She adds that "Zack often turns down work to go to the track, and he's losing clients because of it." Jean admits she did not mind Zack's gambling when they were first married because the bets were small and "it seemed harmless enough." Now, however, "it's like he loves his stupid race-track more than anything, including me."

   Zack admits some concern for his growing debt, "but total payback is only a few good bets away." He also states that "the track gets me away from her nagging." When you see Zack individually, he reveals that he primarily wants to "stay married for my boy, so he can have a dad around." When you ask him for other reasons, he laughs and says, "Well, it can't be for sex. Women can't resist me." He further explains that his "crazy hours" (e.g., often recording all night) enable him to "pick up girls all the time, and Jean just figures I worked late. And if she's not asking, I'm not telling!" He specifically reports having "one-night stands" with "different girls I meet about once a week." Zack acknowledges some fears "about AIDS, but it's too hard to pass up a pretty girl." When you ask why he ever married, he explains, "I thought it would be nice to have someone there for me all the time, and I thought it might be fun to have my own kids."

Clinical Presentation

Zack and Jean are neatly dressed and groomed, alert, and articulate. When you see them together, Zack does most of the talking and often does not let Jean finish her sentences. He seems to be trying to look nonchalant, but he actually appears uncomfortable and somewhat guarded. He maintains this demeanor when he sees you individually. In contrast, Jean is quiet with Zack present, and she appears tense. When you see her alone, however, she is quite verbal but also cries as she recounts her concerns.

   During your conjoint interview, you notice that Jean is wearing a long-sleeve blouse and sweater, even though the weather does not require it. You also notice a black eye and bruises on her left cheek. When you ask her how she got the bruises, Zack quickly states, "She tripped and fell in the backyard, landing on the sprinkler I forgot to put away. I feel just awful about it." Jean simply nods her head in agreement. (The day after your session, however, she calls you from work and says that she had not tripped but that Zack had hit her. Furthermore, he has reportedly "roughed me up" several times in the past 6 months, leaving bruises on her face and arms. She adds that "this is another reason I want counseling, but Zack doesn't want me to tell you. I'd like to leave him, but I don't know where I'd go.")

Assessment Assumptions

No substance abuse or child abuse is present. All factors not explicitly mentioned above have been ruled out. In your waiting room, Zack and Jean each independently completed the Dyadic Adjustment Scale (Spanier 1976). Their scores were both 3 standard deviations below the mean, suggesting a markedly poor relationship.

> **DSM-IV Axis I diagnosis:** 312.31 Pathological gambling
> **DSM-IV Axis II diagnosis:** V71.09 None, narcissistic traits

Identify the impairments and rate their severities on the next page.

The Patient Impairment Profile   93

Steps 1 & 2:
Identifying Impairments and Rating Severity

Instructions: *List **all the impairments,** with their respective **severity ratings.** After each, cite **behavioral evidence (statements/actions)** that supports your choices of both impairments and severities. List the impairments that refer **only to Zack.** Remember that information **not** mentioned should be assumed to be **nonapplicable** to this patient (e.g., no organic pathology is present). Assume that all symptoms and/or relevant information are reported in the case description.*

Impairment Inventory	
Impairment	**Severity rating**
1.	
Behavioral evidence:	
2.	
Behavioral evidence:	
3.	
Behavioral evidence:	
4.	
Behavioral evidence:	
5.	
Behavioral evidence:	

Turn the page for Impairment Inventory and severity rating answers.

Impairment Inventory	
(Impairments are listed chronologically as they appear in the vignette.)	
Impairment	**Severity rating**
1. Physical Abuse Perpetrator *(critical)*	**3** *(Severely incapacitating)*
Behavioral evidence: Zack's wife is wearing long sleeves out of season, her face is bruised, and she states that Zack is responsible. The abuse does not appear imminently dangerous, however.	
2. Uncontrolled Gambling *(noncritical)*	**2** *(Destabilizing)*
Behavioral evidence: Zack "goes to the track all the time" and is "always trying to win back his losses." He states, "little bets aren't fun anymore." His gambling is causing harm ($9,000 debt, with court-ordered garnishment of paychecks) and often interferes with work.	
3. Marital/Relationship Dysfunction *(noncritical)*	**2** *(Destabilizing)*
Behavioral evidence: Jean "was actually packing" when Zack agreed to see a "counselor." He talks over Jean in session, finishing her sentences. He admits having sex often with other women without Jean's knowing. Jean feels " he loves his stupid racetrack more than me." She would "like to leave him." Their scores on the Dyadic Adjustment Scale were both 3 standard deviations below the mean, suggesting a markedly poor relationship.	
4. Promiscuity *(noncritical)*	**2** *(Destabilizing)*
Behavioral evidence: Zack states that he has "one-night stands" with "different girls I meet about once a week." He acknowledges some fears "about AIDS, but it's too hard to pass up a pretty girl."	
5. Egocentricity *(noncritical)*	**2** *(Destabilizing)*
Behavioral evidence: Zack shows empathic failure (e.g., he laughs about infidelity), is arrogant (e.g., "Women can't resist me."), and evaluates primarily in self-centered terms (e.g., "*my* boy," "I thought it would be nice to have someone there for me all the time....I thought it might be fun to have *my* own kids.")	

Common Errors

Assaultiveness: Zack has reportedly assaulted his wife on several occasions. This behavior is already addressed, however, by his Physical Abuse Perpetrator impairment. Remember that *strict adherence to the operational definitions is essential to ensure reliability, for the purpose of communication via the PIP.*

Lying: Some clinicians might identify this impairment because Zack reports having multiple sexual encounters, "and Jean just figures I worked late." However, he is not engaging in deliberate "repetitive falsification." Rather, he is simply not telling his wife, who apparently chooses not to ask. This might reflect Inadequate Self-Maintenance Skills (e.g., pathological dependency) on her part.

Create the Patient Impairment Profile (PIP) on the next page.

The Patient Impairment Profile

Step 3: Creating the Patient Impairment Profile

Instructions: *Now, select those impairments from Zack's Impairment Inventory that will be the current focus of treatment. List them with their respective severity ratings on the Patient Impairment Profile below. List the impairments in **prioritized order.** Then, in the space below, write your rationale for your ranking of each. Remember that information **not** mentioned should be assumed to be **nonapplicable** to this patient.*

Patient Impairment Profile	
Impairment	**Severity rating**
1.	
2.	
3.	
4.	
5.	

1. Prioritization rationale:

2. Prioritization rationale:

3. Prioritization rationale:

4. Prioritization rationale:

5. Prioritization rationale:

Turn the page for prioritized PIP answers.

96   Casebook for Managing Managed Care

Case Presentation 14: Zack Patient Impairment Profile	
Impairment	**Severity rating**
1. Physical Abuse Perpetrator	3
2. Promiscuity	2
3. Uncontrolled Gambling	2
4. Egocentricity	2
5. Marital/Relationship Dysfunction	2

1. Prioritization rationale: Because Zack's behavior represents potential danger to his wife, this severely incapacitating (severity of 3) treatment concern must receive top priority.

2. Prioritization rationale: Treatment of this destabilizing impairment (severity of 2) will have major ramifications for Zack's marriage. Even if the marriage dissolves, however, his Promiscuity still merits treatment. Furthermore, if it is associated with severely incapacitating (severity of 3) Inadequate Healthcare Skills (e.g., lack of condom use), then this latter impairment will need to be added to Zack's PIP.

3. Prioritization rationale: This destabilizing impairment (severity of 2) is also exacerbating the Marital/Relationship Dysfunction (e.g., Jean feels that "he loves his stupid racetrack more than me."). In addition, if Zack continues to accrue debt, his gambling might also provide the basis for assigning Inadequate Self-Maintenance Skills as an additional impairment.

4. Prioritization rationale: This destabilizing impairment (severity of 2) also requires attention whether or not Zack's marriage continues. Treatment might focus on increasing empathy and helping him to develop a more realistic perspective regarding individual and interpersonal issues.

5. Prioritization rationale: If Zack does actually want his marital relationship to improve, this destabilizing (severity of 2) impairment must be addressed. Treatment might begin by further assessing both partners' strongly expressed ambivalence about the marriage (e.g., Zack's Promiscuity and Jean's desire "to leave him").

Common Error

Marital/Relationship Dysfunction: Because all of Zack's impairments except Physical Abuse Perpetrator have the same severity, some clinicians might assign second priority to his Marital/Relationship Dysfunction. Indeed, Zack did cite marriage problems as his reason for seeking

The Patient Impairment Profile

treatment. However, Zack's other destabilizing impairments represent valid treatment foci *whether or not* the marriage dissolves. Furthermore Zack's Promiscuity, Uncontrolled Gambling, and Egocentricity all have direct effects on his marriage as well. Note that *the patient's perspective clearly influences construction of the PIP, but prioritization of the impairments is ultimately the clinician's responsibility.*

Notes

Turn the page for the next case.

Case Presentation 15

"Dean"

Reason for Referral

Dean, a 32-year-old Caucasian man, was referred to you by a hospital social worker. The prior evening, Dean was admitted to the locked psychiatric unit, following a week-long "buying spree" during which he charged $4,000 worth of expensive clothes on his credit card. During this same period, he states that he "drove around about 14 hours a day" and "only got about 3 hours of sleep" per night over the entire week. After Dean was stopped for speeding (at 90 mph and wearing no seat belt), the police brought him to the hospital for an evaluation. Records indicate that this is his first hospitalization. You interview Dean in his hospital room and obtain the following information:

History

Dean is a manager at a 24-hour fast-food restaurant. Two months ago, he began working the graveyard shift. He lives alone, has several friends, and has no history of psychiatric treatment. He supplements his income with a small business (selling mail-order household goods). He says his life has been "pretty average until lately." Over the past few weeks, he reports, "Things have changed beyond my wildest hopes, and I have been able to think of literally thousands of ways to make my business take off!" Dean began spending less time sleeping because "I needed to work on my business ideas, and I wasn't tired anyway." His friends began to notice behavior changes (which became increasingly apparent) several weeks ago. He drove many hours a day "to shop or find new customers who would buy my products." Dean states, "I have felt really energetic a few times in the past, and my friends couldn't believe how 'up' I was, but it's never been this fantastic!" Initially, his increased energy resulted in a measurable improvement in his mail-order business. However, he admits that more recently he has also felt increasingly irritable, especially when managing the restaurant. "My friends at work started complaining I'm getting too intense, but they should remember I'm their boss, too! I don't have to take anything from anybody!"

According to hospital records, Dean was started on lithium immediately on admission; however, he developed a very painful discoloration and coldness in his fingers and toes (resembling Raynaud's disease). The lithium was discontinued, and an alternative medication regimen has just been initiated. At present, Dean is not suicidal, but he is on a locked unit for his protection based on his erratic behavior.

Clinical Presentation

Dean presents as a casually groomed, slightly disheveled man of average height and weight. He is alert, coherent, generally very pleasant, and extremely talkative. He feels challenged when interrupted. Dean incessantly pesters you to look at his mail-order catalog and consider making a purchase. He quickly becomes quite irritated whenever you state that this would not be appropriate. When you ask him how he is feeling right now, he abruptly resumes his pleasant demeanor and replies, "I feel okay except for my fingers and toes! They say it's a reaction to that first medicine, and I don't really think I need this new medicine either, but I guess all those doctors can't be wrong!"

Assessment Assumptions

No hallucinations or delusions and no substance abuse is present. All factors not explicitly mentioned above have been ruled out.

> **DSM-IV Axis I diagnosis**: 296.03 Bipolar I disorder, single manic episode
> **DSM-IV Axis II diagnosis:** None

Identify the impairments and rate their severities on the next page.

The Patient Impairment Profile

Steps 1 & 2:
Identifying Impairments and Rating Severity

Instructions: *List **all the impairments,** with their respective **severity ratings.** After each, cite **behavioral evidence (statements/actions)** that supports your choices of both impairments and severities. List the impairments that refer **only to Dean.** Remember that information **not** mentioned should be assumed to be **nonapplicable** to this patient (e.g., no organic pathology is present). Assume that all symptoms and/or relevant information are reported in the case description.*

Impairment Inventory	
Impairment	**Severity rating**
1.	
Behavioral evidence:	
2.	
Behavioral evidence:	
3.	
Behavioral evidence:	
4.	
Behavioral evidence:	
5.	
Behavioral evidence:	

Turn the page for Impairment Inventory and severity rating answers.

Impairment Inventory	
(Impairments are listed chronologically as they appear in the vignette.)	
Impairment	**Severity rating**
1. Uncontrolled Buying *(noncritical)*	**2** *(Destabilizing)*
Behavioral evidence: During a week-long period, Dean reportedly spent $4,000 with his credit card buying expensive clothes.	
2. Altered Sleep *(noncritical)*	**2** *(Destabilizing)*
Behavioral evidence: During the past week, Dean reports getting "about 3 hours of sleep" per night. Over the past 2 months, he has been spending less time sleeping because "I needed to work on my business ideas, and I wasn't tired anyway."	
3. Manic Thought/Behavior *(critical)*	**4** *(Imminently dangerous)*
Behavioral evidence: Dean states, "I have been able to think of literally thousands of ways to make my business take off!" Recently, he "drove around about 14 hours a day" and "only got about 3 hours of sleep" per night. He has placed himself and others in imminent danger by reckless driving (90 mph with no seat belt). Current hospital records continue to describe his behavior as erratic.	
4. Medical Risk Factor *(critical)*	**2** *(Destabilizing)*
Behavioral evidence: Dean began receiving lithium immediately after his admission, but this treatment caused him to develop very painful discoloration and coldness in his fingers and toes (resembling Raynaud's disease).	

Common Errors

Motor Hyperactivity: Dean's pattern of speech might be considered to represent "actions that are performed at a greater than normal rate of speed," but he demonstrates no hyperactive movements and is not "constantly restless and in motion." In addition, the Impairment Lexicon distinguishes between Manic Thought/Behavior and Motor Hyperactivity. Remember that *strict adherence to the operational definitions is essential to ensure reliability, for the purpose of communication via the PIP.*

Egocentricity: Whereas Dean does show "excessive self-importance," it is also grandiose (e.g., he thinks of "thousands" of business ideas, and he does not "have to take anything from anybody!"). Furthermore, the Impairment Lexicon also distinguishes between Manic Thought/Behavior and Egocentricity, once again showing the importance of *strict adherence to the operational definitions.*

Create the Patient Impairment Profile (PIP) on the next page.

The Patient Impairment Profile

Step 3: Creating the Patient Impairment Profile

Instructions: *Now, select those impairments from Dean's Impairment Inventory that will be the current focus of treatment. List them with their respective severity ratings on the Patient Impairment Profile below. List the impairments in **prioritized order.** Then, in the space below, write your rationale for your ranking of each. Remember that information **not** mentioned should be assumed to be **nonapplicable** to this patient.*

Patient Impairment Profile	
Impairment	**Severity rating**
1.	
2.	
3.	
4.	

1. Prioritization rationale:

2. Prioritization rationale:

3. Prioritization rationale:

4. Prioritization rationale:

Turn the page for prioritized PIP answers.

Case Presentation 15: Dean Patient Impairment Profile	
Impairment	**Severity rating**
1. Manic Thought/Behavior	4
2. Medical Risk Factor	2
3. Altered Sleep	2

1. Prioritization rationale: Dean's safety must be ensured (locked unit) while attempting to stabilize this imminently dangerous (severity of 4) impairment. Once he is stabilized, treatment might focus on helping him cope with the sequelae of his condition (e.g., his need for medication, his credit card bill, and his strained relationships with friends and co-workers). Uncontrolled Buying should spontaneously remit as behavioral evidence of improvement regarding his Manic Thought/Behavior.

2. Prioritization rationale: An appropriate medication protocol (i.e., one that does not adversely affect Dean but does control his symptoms) must be established to eliminate this destabilizing (severity of 2) impairment.

3. Prioritization rationale: Whether Dean's Altered Sleep over the past 2 months was caused entirely by his Manic Thought/Behavior or whether the former preceded the onset of the latter is unclear. Thus, additional assessment of this destabilizing (severity of 2) impairment is warranted, the results of which will determine further treatment decisions.

Common Error

Uncontrolled Buying: Given the serious nature of this impairment (i.e., that it involved charging $4,000 for clothing in 1 week), some clinicians might include it in the PIP. However, Dean's Uncontrolled Buying apparently was due to—and occurred entirely within the context of—his Manic Thought/Behavior. As such, effective treatment of the latter should cause spontaneous remission of the former. Remember to *avoid "stuffing" a PIP with tangential or redundant impairments.*

Goals and Objectives
Performance Measures for Managed Care

In this chapter, we illustrate how the Patient Impairment Profile (PIP) is used as a basis for determining the goals of treatment, as well as the objectives signaling progress toward these goals. Two cases covered earlier in this book are used to illustrate this process. Then two new cases are presented, providing the reader opportunity to develop additional PIPs and study their links to goals and objectives.

Definitions

outcome measure   An indicator (performance measure) that captures and quantifies the results of care.

patient objective   An anticipated patient statement or behavior that shows progress toward repair of an impairment.

target objective   An anticipated patient statement or behavior that signals "discharge" to less service-intensive treatment.

treatment goal   The repair of an impairment or reduction in severity of an impairment to a treatment endpoint. Attaining *endpoint goals* marks the completion of treatment. Treatment involving transition from one level of care to another can include an *interim goal* that signals this transition. For patients requiring intermittent and/or ongoing care, treatment can involve *maintenance goals*.

Many different approaches can be taken to ascertain *treatment goals* and patient objectives. With the PIP, however, goals are determined by simple logic. Specifically, goals always involve *the repair of an impairment (severity of 0) or reduction in severity of an impairment to a treatment endpoint*. Thus, for each impairment cited in the PIP, one goal naturally follows.

Progress toward treatment goals is measured in two ways: 1) by the degree of reduction in initial severity ratings and 2) by *patient objectives,* which are anticipated patient statements or behaviors (actions) that indicate progress toward repair of an impairment. Basing objectives on quantifiable information (e.g., standardized *outcome measures)* can also be helpful in documenting progress to reviewers (see Chapter 7), particularly regarding small changes. Doing so, however, necessitates that reviewers and clinicians are both able to interpret test results appropriately, with special attention given to reliability and validity issues (Nunnally and Bernstein 1994). A wide variety of such measures, many focusing on specific problem areas, are readily available (e.g., Fischer and Corcoran 1994a, 1994b).

When dealing with transitions from more intensive treatment settings (e.g., hospitalization) to less intensive ones (e.g., day treatment center), *target objectives* are identified. A target objective is an anticipated patient statement or behavior that signals "discharge" to less service-intensive treatment. In turn, *interim goals* are logically accomplished by attaining all target objectives.

April's Treatment Goals and Patient Objectives
(Case 11 continued)

Because of the imminently dangerous nature of April's Psychotic Thought/Behavior, she was placed in a locked psychiatric inpatient unit. Based on her long-term history, she will presumably require continued care after hospital discharge. Thus, the initial goals set forth are *interim goals* to be met prior to her transition to a less restrictive/intensive treatment setting. The following are *suggestions* only.

Case Presentation 11: April (see Chapter 4) Patient Impairment Profile		
	Severity rating .	
Impairment	**4/10/2001**	**Interim goal**
1. Delusions (Nonparanoid)	4	2
2. Psychotic Thought/Behavior	3	2
3. Inadequate Self-Maintenance Skills	2	1
4. Educational Performance Deficit	2	2

For April, target objectives needed to be identified that—when accomplished (100%)—would signal her completion of *interim goals* and her readiness to progress to a less service-intensive treatment and resume optimal functioning. Given the long-term nature of her illness, it was assumed that treatment would culminate in her achieving *maintenance goals*. (In contrast, a short-term patient's goals would presumably be *endpoint goals,* involving the complete *repair* of impairments.)

Goals and Objectives

Given the working assumption that her rapid deterioration was caused by an excessive decrease in her medication levels, a short inpatient treatment would focus primarily on reestablishing therapeutic medication levels. The following initial objectives are *suggestions* only:

Case Presentation 11: April (continued)

Patient Objectives

To Be Addressed by Discharge From Inpatient Setting to Group Home Setting: 4/16/2001

(*Target Objective—to be met 100%)

Delusions (Nonparanoid)

Patient will verbalize
- Awareness of the presence of delusional thinking
- Acceptance of the responsibility for coping with the Delusions
- Precipitants for the delusional thinking
- Warning signs that the Delusions are exacerbating
- * A plan of action to be taken should the Delusions exacerbate

Patient will demonstrate
- * Absence of Delusions for 72 hours
- Adherence to prescribed treatment program
- * A completed self-care (discharge) plan, including steps to be taken should the Delusions return or exacerbate

Psychotic Thought/Behavior

Patient will verbalize
- Awareness of the presence of Psychotic Thought/Behavior
- Acceptance of the responsibility for coping with the Psychotic Thought/Behavior
- Precipitants for the Psychotic Thought/Behavior
- Warning signs that the Psychotic Thought/Behavior is exacerbating
- * A plan of action to be taken should the Psychotic Thought/Behavior exacerbate

Patient will demonstrate
- * Absence of Psychotic Thought/Behavior for 72 hours
- Adherence to prescribed treatment program
- * A completed self-care (discharge) plan, including steps to be taken should the Psychotic Thought/Behavior return or exacerbate

(continued)

To Be Addressed by Completion of Treatment and Resumption of Semi-Independent Living: 6/18/2001

Delusions (Nonparanoid)

Patient will verbalize
- Awareness that Delusions can resume without maintained adherence to discharge plan

Patient will demonstrate
- Maintained adherence to self-care plan with maintained absence of Delusions

Psychotic Thought/Behavior

Patient will verbalize
- Awareness that Psychotic Thought/Behavior can resume without maintained adherence to discharge plan

Patient will demonstrate
- Maintained adherence to self-care plan with adequate management of Psychotic Thought/Behavior

Inadequate Self-Maintenance Skills

Patient will verbalize
- Awareness of the presence of Inadequate Self-Maintenance Skills
- Acceptance of the responsibility for coping with the Inadequate Self-Maintenance Skills
- Awareness of the dangers or adverse consequences of Inadequate Self-Maintenance Skills
- A plan of action to be taken should the Inadequate Self-Maintenance Skills exacerbate

Patient will demonstrate
- Adherence to a prescribed treatment program
- Adequate management of the Inadequate Self-Maintenance Skills
- A completed self-care (discharge) plan, including steps to be taken should the Inadequate Self-Maintenance Skills return or exacerbate

Educational Performance Deficit

Patient will verbalize
- Awareness of the Educational Performance Deficit and its negative effect
- Acceptance of the responsibility for coping with the Educational Performance Deficit
- Willingness to participate in an Educational Performance Deficit assessment and remediation program

Patient will demonstrate
- Participation in a remediation program

Goals and Objectives

Because it is clearly desirable for all of a patient's impairments to be repaired completely, it is logical to set optimal goals and objectives initially. As treatment continues, behaviorally supported (statements/actions) realistic constraints to progress can be documented as justification for the clinical necessity of additional treatment and/or the need to replace an *endpoint goal* with a *maintenance goal*. For example, intelligence and achievement assessment might reveal that April's Educational Performance Deficit is not remediable, in which case related goals and objectives will need to be altered.

Billy's Treatment Goals and Patient Objectives
(Case 12 continued)

Aside from Billy's "failure to develop full nocturnal bladder control," he is apparently a generally well-adjusted little boy with well-adjusted parents. Thus, his needs for treatment were viewed as straight-forward. Once-weekly family therapy was prescribed, and the initial goals were also viewed as the endpoint goals of treatment. The following goals are *suggestions* only:

Case Presentation 12: Billy (see Chapter 4)		
Patient Impairment Profile		
	Severity rating	
Impairment	**7/2/2001**	**Endpoint goal**
1. Enuresis	1	0
2. Pathological Guilt	1	0

Billy's treatment is not expected to involve any transitions between treatment settings, so no objectives are identified as target objectives. Instead, the completion of all objectives will signal the accomplishment of all treatment goals (i.e., the total *repair* of all impairments). The following patient objectives are *suggestions* only:

Case Presentation 12: Billy (continued)
Patient Objectives
To Be Addressed by Treatment Completion: 8/13/2001
Enuresis
Patient will verbalize
• Awareness of the presence of Enuresis
• Acceptance of the responsibility for coping with the Enuresis
• Willingness to participate in the treatment of Enuresis
• A plan of action to be taken should the Enuresis exacerbate
(continued)

Patient will demonstrate

- Adherence to a prescribed treatment program
- Elimination of Enuresis
- A completed self-care (discharge) plan, including steps to be taken should the Enuresis exacerbate

Pathological Guilt

Patient will verbalize

- Awareness of the Pathological Guilt and its current adverse consequences (e.g., generalized anxiety)
- Willingness to participate in the treatment of Pathological Guilt

Patient will demonstrate

- Elimination of Pathological Guilt as evidenced by cessation of repetitive apologizing behavior
- A completed self-care (discharge) plan, including steps to be taken should the Pathological Guilt exacerbate

The clinician may question whether our frequently suggested initial objective, involving "acceptance of the responsibility for coping with" an impairment, may be compared with counterproductive self-blame. Billy's case illustrates that such a comparison is inappropriate. Clearly, no clinician would want Billy to increase his self-blame for Enuresis because such behavior is the basis of his Pathological Guilt. In contrast, "acceptance of responsibility" is intended to be viewed as an empowering preliminary step toward resolving a personal problem. Conversely, failure to accept responsibility can be equated with viewing an impairment as out of one's control, rendering any proposed intervention as unfeasible and promoting feelings of hopelessness. In Billy's case, "accepting responsibility" would involve clarifying that no one thought he wet the bed intentionally and that bed-wetting is not the same as "doing something wrong." Thus, accepting responsibility would actually involve *reduction* of pejorative self-blame. At the same time, however, it would involve empowering Billy to view bed-wetting as a controllable problem that *he could resolve* with the clinician's help.

Step 4: Identifying Goals and Objectives

Two new cases follow. As in Chapter 4, you will create an Impairment Inventory (Steps 1 and 2) and then construct a PIP (Step 3) for each. Although only one set of "correct" impairments is associated with any given case, this is not typically true for treatment goals or patient objectives. The clinician, in collaboration with the patient, makes such decisions. Thus, multiple-choice study questions about goals and objectives are presented to facilitate integration of this new information with previous topics (i.e., impairments, severities, and the PIP). Once again, please read each vignette and imagine that you are actually interviewing the identified patient.

Goals and Objectives

Notes

Turn the page for the next case.

Case Presentation 16
"Lilly"

Reason for Referral

Lilly, a 28-year-old Asian American woman, was self-referred. She called because "I am miserable" and "want help dealing with my husband." She complained that he has been "stingy" about their finances lately, causing considerable strain on their marriage. You interview Lilly and her husband and obtain the following information:

History

Lilly has been married to Paul, a 45-year-old Asian American man, for 6 years; they have no children. Paul is a successful jewelry store owner. They dated for 4 months before getting married. Paul states that "she made me feel 10 years younger back then, but she weighed less and she was nicer to be around." Lilly reports spending most of her time "shopping and trying to enjoy life." They live in a large home in an affluent area.

Paul grew up in a family in which "we had to work hard just to pay the bills." He worked his way through community college (A.A. degree) and then "worked two jobs" for several years to accrue the funds needed to start his business. He then worked 14-hour days for the next several years to pay off his loans. When he first met Lilly, Paul had been debt-free for only 2 years, having sacrificed much of his social life to accomplish this.

Lilly was an only child of wealthy parents who gave her whatever she wanted. She attended boarding school from sixth grade on but resumed living at home after high school. She began college several times but never finished. At age 22, she moved into her own townhouse in an exclusive neighborhood, at which time her mother experienced major depression for "about 6 months." Lilly worked sporadically for her father but never sought work elsewhere. After marrying (which disappointed her parents), she quit her job. Paul's business success during the first 3 years enabled them to maintain the lifestyle to which Lilly had been accustomed. When business slowed, however, he started complaining about her spending. This hurt Lilly, and Paul describes the 2 years since then as "murder, because she is always down about one thing or another." Lilly admits, "I feel like crying most days and I've been eating more, but how can I feel good at all when Paul doesn't show his love? A woman needs to know she is loved!" Recently, Paul has begun to pressure Lilly to "get a job and earn her keep," but she protests, "I'm too tired most days to go out, let alone work! If he were a better businessman, there would be no problem."

Paul is concerned by the growing debt. He complains, "I try to please her, but she is never happy, and I can never do enough. Everything is my fault." He continues, "If I want any sex, she's got to get whatever she wants, and she dresses too sexy when she goes out."

Clinical Presentation

Lilly is slightly overweight and immaculately dressed and groomed, wearing a short skirt, low-cut blouse, and gold jewelry. She pulls her chair closer to yours, slightly in front of Paul. Her demeanor is seductive. She is coherent, but her speech (e.g., her complaints) lacks detail (e.g., "he is so stingy," "he's just not the same") and is generally self-focused (e.g., "I" versus "we"). Her emotional expression appears theatrically exaggerated and is predominantly sad but also changes quickly (e.g., crying in response to mildly emotional issues, laughing in response to her own joke). She often explains her problems in terms of what Paul is or is not doing, and she shows little concern when you ask how she thinks he feels. Paul is short, bald, well dressed and groomed, and of average weight. He appears sullen, often rolling his eyes in response to Lilly and saying little. When he tries to assert himself, Lilly talks over him and he acquiesces.

Assessment Assumptions

No substance abuse is present, and Paul's perspective is generally accurate. All factors not explicitly mentioned above have been ruled out. In your waiting room, Lilly completed the Center for Epidemiologic Studies—Depressed Mood Scale (Radloff 1977) and the Index of Marital Satisfaction (Hudson 1992). Both scores were more than 3 standard deviations from the mean, reflecting marked symptomatology.

> **Important note:** For this case, presume you are a *male* therapist.
>
> **DSM-IV Axis I diagnosis:** 300.4 Dysthymic disorder
> **DSM-IV Axis II diagnosis:** 301.50 Histrionic personality disorder
>
> *Identify the impairments and rate their severities on the next page.*

Goals and Objectives   **111**

Steps 1 & 2:
Identifying Impairments and Rating Severity

Instructions: *List **all the impairments,** with their respective **severity ratings.** After each, cite **behavioral evidence (statements/actions)** that supports your choices of both impairments and severities. List the impairments that refer **only to Lilly**. Remember that information **not** mentioned should be assumed to be **nonapplicable** to this patient (e.g., no organic pathology is present). Assume that all symptoms and/or relevant information are reported in the case description.*

Impairment Inventory	
Impairment	**Severity rating**
1.	
Behavioral evidence:	
2.	
Behavioral evidence:	
3.	
Behavioral evidence:	
4.	
Behavioral evidence:	
5.	
Behavioral evidence:	

Turn the page for Impairment Inventory and severity rating answers.

Impairment Inventory	
(Impairments are listed chronologically as they appear in the vignette.)	
Impairment	**Severity rating**
1. Dysphoric Mood *(critical)*	**2** *(Destabilizing)*
Behavioral evidence: Lilly is "miserable," and for 2 years, she has been "always down about one thing or another." She feels "like crying most days" and claims she is "too tired most days to go out," yet she spends most of her time "shopping and trying to enjoy life." Her score on the Center for Epidemiologic Studies—Depressed Mood Scale is more than 3 standard deviations above the mean, reflecting marked symptomatology.	
2. Marital/Relationship Dysfunction *(noncritical)*	**2** *(Destabilizing)*
Behavioral evidence: She wants you to "help me deal with my husband." The last 2 years have been "murder." Lilly feels that "Paul doesn't show his love." Paul feels "she is never happy and I can never do enough." When he tries to assert himself, Lilly talks over him and he acquiesces. Her score on the Index of Marital Satisfaction is more than 3 standard deviations below the mean, reflecting marked dissatisfaction. (Paul's Index of Marital Satisfaction score is 1.5 standard deviations below the mean.)	
3. Egocentricity *(noncritical)*	**2** *(Destabilizing)*
Behavioral evidence: She uses self-focused (e.g., "I" versus "we") language, typically "talks over" Paul, and shows little empathy for his feelings. Paul states, "I try to please her...but I can never do enough."	
4. Externalization and Blame *(noncritical)*	**2** *(Destabilizing)*
Behavioral evidence: She explains her problems in terms of what Paul is or is not doing (e.g., "If he were a better businessman, there would be no problem."). Paul says that Lilly thinks "everything is my fault."	
5. Manipulativeness *(noncritical)*	**1** *(Distressing)*
Behavioral evidence: Paul reports, "If I want any sex, she's got to get whatever she wants." She positions her chair closer to yours, in front of Paul's, during the session.	

Common Errors

Inadequate Self-Maintenance Skills: Although Lilly might be seen as "pathologically dependent" on Paul, her "dependency" appears to be more a product of her impairments listed above. Even more important, her self-maintenance skills do not "compromise or endanger" her quality of life, which is—in fact—affluent.

Mood Lability: Lilly's *apparent* mood changes seem to be the result of her emotional expression being "theatrically exaggerated" rather than the result of actual "fluctuations...to euphoric or dysphoric states." Furthermore, she is "predominantly sad."

Create the Patient Impairment Profile (PIP) on the next page.

Goals and Objectives

Step 3: Creating the Patient Impairment Profile

Instructions: *Now, select those impairments from Lilly's Impairment Inventory that will be the current focus of treatment. List them with their respective severity ratings on the Patient Impairment Profile below. List the impairments in **prioritized order.** Then, in the space below, write your rationale for your ranking of each. Remember that information **not** mentioned should be assumed to be **nonapplicable** to this patient.*

Patient Impairment Profile	
Impairment	**Severity rating**
1.	
2.	
3.	
4.	
5.	

1. Prioritization rationale:

2. Prioritization rationale:

3. Prioritization rationale:

4. Prioritization rationale:

5. Prioritization rationale:

Turn the page for prioritized PIP answers.

Case Presentation 16: Lilly **Patient Impairment Profile**	
Impairment	**Severity rating**
1. Dysphoric Mood	2
2. Egocentricity	2
3. Externalization and Blame	2
4. Marital/Relationship Dysfunction	2

1. Prioritization rationale: This destabilizing impairment (severity of 2) appears to be exacerbating the Marital/Relationship Dysfunction and appears to be long-standing. It might deter treatment of other problems if not given top priority.

2. Prioritization rationale: Narcissistic perspective and behavior also appear to be destabilizing (severity of 2) Lilly's relationships. Empathy development also might help her marriage.

3. Prioritization rationale: Without learning to accept responsibility, Lilly's ability to initiate behavioral changes will remain destabilized (severity of 2).

4. Prioritization rationale: Lilly also has some destabilizing (severity of 2) relationship problems, but they are not likely to be addressed effectively unless she makes significant progress individually. Treatment might focus on increasing cooperation and improving Paul's assertiveness. Lilly's Manipulativeness seems limited to this realm and as such could be one focus of marital work.

Common Error

Marital/Relationship Dysfunction: This case clearly involves marital issues requiring attention, and marital therapy would certainly be an appropriate primary treatment modality. As such, some clinicians may want to rate Marital/Relationship Dysfunction first in the PIP. Note, however, that Lilly has other impairments with equally great severity ratings. Also note that the PIP does not reflect a *sequence* of treatment issues, as though the first impairment must be addressed and resolved before the next is treated. Rather, the PIP reflects a *prioritization* of impairments that are *concurrent* treatment foci. Thus, marital therapy could be an appropriate primary treatment modality in this case, even though Marital/Relationship Dysfunction appears last in the PIP. If it were the *sole* modality, however, marital therapy also would need to directly address Lilly's other impairments. If this did not seem feasible to the clinician, additional treatment modalities (e.g., individual psychotherapy, psychopharmacotherapy) would need to be proposed (see Chapter 6).

Goals and Objectives

Notes

Turn the page for more on Lilly's case.

Lilly's Treatment Goals and Patient Objectives

Lilly's Axis II diagnosis might render her "untreatable" according to many managed care standards. Thus, her case illustrates the particular utility of the PIP in communicating viable reasons for treatment to reviewers. Note that no term in the Impairment Lexicon describes a "characterological problem," as the recalcitrance of Axis II disorders is well known. As such, the goals of Lilly's treatment will not directly address her histrionic personality disorder. Instead, every impairment in her PIP describes a valid reason for treatment.

Because of the large number of interrelated impairments, multiple intervention modalities were used. Prozac (fluoxetine 20 mg/day) was prescribed for her dysphoric mood, given her family history, complaints of low energy, irritability, and rejection sensitivity. (Furthermore, Prozac should not exacerbate weight gain.) The clinician also used both marital and individual psychotherapy. Specifically, individual and marital sessions were conducted on alternate weeks, resulting in weekly outpatient visits. The following objectives are *suggestions* only:

Case Presentation 16: Lilly		
Patient Impairment Profile		
	Severity rating	
Impairment	**2/26/2001**	**Endpoint goal**
1. Dysphoric Mood	2	0
2. Egocentricity	2	0
3. Externalization and Blame	2	0
4. Marital/Relationship Dysfunction	2	0

Patient Objectives

To Be Addressed by Treatment Completion: 5/7/2001

Dysphoric Mood

Patient will verbalize
- Acceptance of the responsibility for coping with the Dysphoric Mood
- Awareness of the precipitants of negative mood changes
- Statements about self that are realistically positive and hopeful rather than unrealistically negative
- Plans and activities to be initiated with husband or friends
- Warning signs that the Dysphoric Mood is exacerbating
- A plan of action to be taken should the Dysphoric Mood exacerbate

(continued)

Goals and Objectives

Patient will demonstrate
- Adherence to the prescribed treatment program
- Increased self-initiated and self-directed activities
- Elimination of Dysphoric Mood as evidenced by a normal range score on the Center for Epidemiologic Studies—Depressed Mood Scale
- A completed self-care (discharge) plan, including steps to be taken should the Dysphoric Mood return or exacerbate

Egocentricity

Patient will verbalize
- Acceptance of the responsibility for coping with the Egocentricity
- Awareness of the precipitants of egocentric behavior
- Statements that show empathic understanding
- Warning signs that Egocentricity is exacerbating
- A plan of action to be taken should the Egocentricity exacerbate

Patient will demonstrate
- Participation in the prescribed treatment program
- Increased cooperative and decreased demanding behaviors
- Elimination of Egocentricity as evidenced by a normal range score on the Selfism scale (Phares and Erksine 1984)
- A completed self-care (discharge) plan, including steps to be taken should the Egocentricity return or exacerbate

Externalization and Blame

Patient will verbalize
- Acceptance of the responsibility for Externalization and Blame
- Awareness of the precipitants of Externalization and Blame
- Warning signs that Externalization and Blame is exacerbating
- A plan of action to be taken should the Externalization and Blame exacerbate

Patient will demonstrate
- Participation in the prescribed treatment program
- Increased accuracy in identifying her contribution to problems
- Increased ability to admit being wrong and to accept responsibility for behavior
- Elimination of Externalization and Blame
- A completed self-care (discharge) plan, including steps to be taken should the Externalization and Blame return or exacerbate

(continued)

Marital/Relationship Dysfunction

Patient will verbalize
- Acceptance of mutual responsibility for coping with the Marital/Relationship Dysfunction
- Awareness of the precipitants of Marital/Relationship Dysfunction
- Warning signs that Marital/Relationship Dysfunction is worsening
- A plan of action to be taken should the Marital/Relationship Dysfunction exacerbate

Patient will demonstrate
- Participation in the prescribed treatment program
- Ability to identify dysfunctional interpersonal behavior (e.g., manipulation) and correct it
- Ability to discuss and resolve a problem with his or her spouse
- Elimination of Marital/Relationship Dysfunction as evidenced by a normal range score on the Index of Marital Satisfaction.
- A completed self-care (discharge) plan, including steps to be taken should the Marital/Relationship Dysfunction return or exacerbate

Goals and Objectives   **119**

Goals and Objectives:
Study Questions—Lilly

Instructions: *Read each of the questions below and circle the* most *correct response.*

1. The number of treatment goals

   a) is always less than the number of impairments listed in the PIP.
   b) is always greater than the number of impairments listed in the PIP.
   c) is always equivalent to the number of impairments listed in the PIP.
   d) has no correlation with the number of impairments listed in the PIP.

2. Lilly's goal for each impairment in her PIP is a severity of 0. This implies that

   a) the clinician is sure that Lilly will be completely free of all impairments by treatment comple-
      tion on 5/7/2001.
   b) the clinician believes it is appropriate to facilitate Lilly's attempts to resolve all
      impairments completely by 5/7/2001.
   c) the clinician knows that none of Lilly's impairments are chronic.
   d) the clinician assumes that Lilly's problems are uncomplicated and should require minimal
      treatment.

3. If Lilly accomplishes all of the patient objectives for any one impairment, this implies that

   a) she is well on her way to repairing that impairment.
   b) she is well on her way to completing treatment.
   c) treatment has resulted in repair of that impairment.
   d) it is impossible for that impairment to reappear later in her PIP.

4. Lilly's patient objectives for Marital/Relationship Dysfunction and her treatment goal for this impairment

   a) can still be met even if her spouse refuses to cooperate.
   b) are totally independent of her other impairments.
   c) will be addressed after her other impairments are repaired.
   d) are contingent for success on her spouse's cooperation.

5. If Lilly obtains a normal range score on the Index of Marital Satisfaction, this implies that

   a) she is currently accomplishing one patient objective toward the treatment goal of eliminating
      her Marital/Relationship Dysfunction.
   b) her Marital/Relationship Dysfunction has been repaired.
   c) she must maintain such a score over time to show that the Marital/Relationship Dysfunction is
      truly repaired.
   d) her marriage is now functioning in an exemplary fashion.

Turn the page for the answers to these questions.

Goals and Objectives:
Answers to Study Questions

1. Answer "c" is correct. The number of treatment goals is always equivalent to the number of impairments listed in the PIP. By definition, a *treatment goal* is the repair of an impairment or reduction in severity of an impairment to an endpoint or maintenance level. Thus, each impairment listed in a PIP mandates one treatment goal.

2. Answer "b" is correct. No transition between treatment settings is anticipated for Lilly. As such, her treatment does not involve any *interim* goals. Because she does not present with a specific history of chronic impairments, it is premature to assume that only *maintenance* goals can be identified. As such, all of Lilly's goals are *endpoint* goals. It is appropriate to assign severities of 0 as endpoint goals at the beginning of treatment, because ethical treatment aims for optimal efficacy. This does not imply that the clinician predicts complete recovery with any degree of certainty (Answer "a") nor does it imply that Lilly's impairments *cannot* turn out to be chronic (Answer "c"). After gathering more data and treating her for some time, the clinician may reassess some of Lilly's impairments to be more long-standing. At such time, treatment goals could be changed to maintenance goals (e.g., severity of 1). Finally, severities of 0 as treatment goals do not imply that problems or treatments are assumed to be simple (Answer "d"). Rather, the ethical clinician will always assign the optimal treatment goal, at least initially, as part of efforts to optimize treatment efficacy.

3. Answer "c" is correct. Beyond being "well on her way" (Answer "a"), Lilly has repaired a given impairment by meeting all of its objectives (including any objectives added subsequent to the initial evaluation). In contrast, repairing one impairment does not automatically imply anything regarding other impairments in a PIP or treatment overall (Answer "b"). Furthermore, meeting an objective—or even all the objectives—for an impairment does not guarantee that it might not reappear (Answer "d"). The PIP is dynamic and can reflect the reemergence of impairments (e.g., with setbacks or with chronic problems).

4. Answer "d" is correct. This question is a bit tricky, because all impairments in the Impairment Lexicon are intended to enable communication about an *individual* identified patient. However, for those impairments describing problems directly involving *other persons* (i.e., Family Dysfunction and Marital/Relationship Dysfunction), it is assumed that a functional relationship is desired. Clearly, healthy relationships necessitate cooperation and motivation from all relevant parties. Thus, this impairment cannot be repaired independently (Answer "a"). Furthermore, an individual wishing to reunite with a former partner *who has no interest to do so* could not even be identified as experiencing this impairment (see "Case Presentation 10: Carlos" in Chapter 3). Answer "b" is incorrect, because impairments rarely occur in a vacuum. Rather, progress with objectives for one impairment will often (but not always) have ramifications for progress on others. Finally, Answer "c" is incorrect, because a PIP never implies sequential treatment of impairments.

5. Answer "a" is correct. Meeting one objective—even if it involves a scale score implying normal function—does not imply total repair of an impairment (Answers "b" and "c"). By definition, total repair involves meeting all objectives. Finally, achieving a normal score typically signifies *average,* not exemplary, functioning (Answer "d"). Exemplary functioning would be associated with a scale score suggesting at least above-average functioning.

Goals and Objectives

Notes

Turn the page for the next case.

Casebook for Managing Managed Care

Case Presentation 17

"Eddie"

Reason for Referral

The P. family has come to your office on the recommendation of the school psychologist. Eddie, an 8-year-old Latino boy, has had a very irregular pattern of school attendance since the school year began 3 months ago. Eddie's teacher reports that his schoolwork is satisfactory when he attends but that his absences result in most of his time being spent "catching up." Eddie is bright, but his teacher fears that he will not be able to stay caught up "because the curriculum really gets more difficult soon." You interview the P. family and obtain the following information:

History

Eddie lives with his mother (age 28), stepfather (age 35), stepsister (age 10), and stepbrother (age 13). (Eddie's father lives out of state and rarely sees him.) His mother reports that she and her husband both feel "children should be in school," but she explains that Eddie often "kicks, screams, fusses, and fights" until she lets him stay home. His "fussing" is not new, but his reluctance to attend school only started this year. Eddie's stepfather believes this might be due to Eddie's "getting in the habit of being with his mom all the time after her surgery this summer." (Eddie's mother had an appendectomy in July, and Eddie became her "little helper" during her recuperation at home.)

Eddie's teacher has noted that when Eddie does come to school, he often complains of headaches or stomachaches and asks to see the nurse. On various occasions, he has been sent home because of this. Mr. and Mrs. P. tell you that he voices the same complaints at home (and/or "throws a fit") whenever his mother tries to go anywhere without him. Eddie's mother admits, "Whenever I try to leave, he asks, 'What if you don't come back'?" Eddie's parents also report taking Eddie to the physician often for his stomachache and headache complaints. The doctor, however, has not found any physical problem and according to Eddie's mother "had the nerve to say it might just be in his head."

Clinical Presentation

Eddie presents as a neatly dressed and groomed, slightly overweight boy of below average height for his age. His speech is normal with coherent content. He appears to be somewhat shy, and early in the session, he complains to his mother that his "stomach hurts." His mother responds by placing Eddie on her lap where he stays for the remainder of the time. After this, Eddie shows no outward signs of distress. He responds to your questions with age-appropriate answers. When asked about his school refusal, he replies, "I'd rather be at home with mom so I can be her helper" and also cites his stomach discomfort.

Eddie's stepfather speaks little, but he occasionally nods in agreement in response to prompts from his wife. He expresses concern for Eddie but explains that his job has kept him away for long hours "to help pay the surgery bills insurance didn't cover." Eddie's mother is quite verbal and maintains good eye contact. Both parents appear genuinely concerned, although there is little direct communication between them.

Assessment Assumptions

No sexual, physical, or emotional abuse is present. All factors not explicitly mentioned above have been ruled out. In your waiting room, Eddie's parents completed the Eyberg Child Behavior Inventory (Burns and Patterson 1990). Eddie's scores were 1.5 standard deviations above the mean, suggesting some behavior problems.

> **DSM-IV Axis I diagnosis:** 309.21 Separation anxiety disorder
> **DSM-IV Axis II diagnosis:** None

Identify the impairments and rate their severities on the next page.

Goals and Objectives   **123**

Steps 1 & 2:
Identifying Impairments and Rating Severity

Instructions: *List **all the impairments,** with their respective **severity ratings.** After each, cite **behavioral evidence (statements/actions)** that supports your choices of both impairments and severities. List the impairments that refer **only to Eddie.** Remember that information **not** mentioned should be assumed to be **nonapplicable** to this patient (e.g., no organic pathology is present). Assume that all symptoms and/or relevant information are reported in the case description.*

Impairment Inventory	
Impairment	**Severity rating**
1.	
Behavioral evidence:	
2.	
Behavioral evidence:	
3.	
Behavioral evidence:	
4.	
Behavioral evidence:	
5.	
Behavioral evidence:	

Turn the page for Impairment Inventory and severity rating answers.

Impairment Inventory *(Impairments are listed chronologically as they appear in the vignette.)*	
Impairment	**Severity rating**
1. School Avoidance *(noncritical)*	**1** *(Distressing)*
Behavioral evidence: Eddie has had very irregular school attendance for 3 months. He "kicks, screams, fusses, and fights" until his mother lets him stay home. He would "rather be at home with mom so I can be her helper."	
2. Somatization *(noncritical)*	**1** *(Distressing)*
Behavioral evidence: At school, he often complains of headaches or stomachaches and asks to see the nurse. He also makes such complaints at home. Frequent trips to the physician have not found any physical problem, and the physician reportedly thinks "it might just be in his head."	
3. Family Dysfunction *(noncritical)*	**1** *(Distressing)*
Behavioral evidence: Mrs. P. lets Eddie stay home from school, where he is her "little helper." When he complains in session that his "stomach hurts," his mother places him on her lap, where he stays. The stepfather seems somewhat disengaged. Little communication occurs between spouses.	
4. Tantrums *(noncritical)*	**2** *(Destabilizing)*
Behavioral evidence: Eddie often "kicks, screams, fusses, and fights" until his mother lets him stay home from school. His "fussing" is not new, and he does it ("throws a fit") whenever his mother tries to go anywhere without him. Eddie's Eyberg Child Behavior Inventory scores were 1.5 standard deviations above the mean, suggesting some behavior problems.	

Common Errors

Anxiety: Eddie does show some "uneasiness...[or]...apprehension," but it appears to be surrounding his School Avoidance. Some clinicians may be tempted to cite Anxiety as a latent impairment. However, impairments by definition are always manifest and behaviorally supportable. Including "assessment for potential Anxiety" as an intervention (see Chapter 6) in connection with his School Avoidance would be appropriate. In addition, Anxiety might emerge in the future as the School Avoidance is corrected. At such time, adding Anxiety to the PIP would be appropriate but not before this (or any) impairment is behaviorally supported.

Manipulativeness: Eddie's Tantrums might be described as manipulative, but the clinical information (e.g., he is only 8 years old) presented does not suggest that he is *intentionally* using Tantrums "solely to gain [his] own ends." The fact that his Tantrums do result in Eddie's getting his way is more likely related to the Family Dysfunction he also experiences.

Create the Patient Impairment Profile (PIP) on the next page.

Goals and Objectives

Step 3: Creating the Patient Impairment Profile

Instructions: *Now, select those impairments from Eddie's Impairment Inventory that will be the current focus of treatment. List them with their respective severity ratings on the Patient Impairment Profile below. List the impairments in **prioritized order.** Then, in the space below, write your rationale for your ranking of each. Remember that information **not** mentioned should be assumed to be **nonapplicable** to this patient.*

Patient Impairment Profile	
Impairment	**Severity rating**
1.	
2.	
3.	
4.	

1. Prioritization rationale:

2. Prioritization rationale:

3. Prioritization rationale:

4. Prioritization rationale:

Turn the page for prioritized PIP answers.

Case Presentation 17: Eddie	
Patient Impairment Profile	
Impairment	**Severity rating**
1. Tantrums	2
2. School Avoidance	1
3. Somatization	1

1. Prioritization rationale: Eddie's Tantrums are "not new," are not limited to his School Avoidance, and are destabilizing (severity of 2) his functioning. Thus, direct treatment of Tantrums is warranted. Family therapy and/or behavior modification might be useful to this end.

2. Prioritization rationale: Distress (severity of 1) caused by Eddie's school absences must be reduced/eliminated before his educational performance is significantly affected.

3. Prioritization rationale: Eddie's distressing (severity of 1) somatic complaints are not limited to his School Avoidance. (He even uses them in the session to get maternal attention.) Thus, they merit direct treatment in their own right.

Note: Eddie's Family Dysfunction appears to be subsumed by his School Avoidance and Tantrums. Additional assessment as treatment progresses might reveal a more pervasive Family Dysfunction. In either case, treatment options might include family therapy.

Common Error

Family Dysfunction: Because this case lends itself well to a family therapy approach, some clinicians might be tempted to enter Family Dysfunction first in the PIP. According to the Impairment Inventory, however, Eddie's Family Dysfunction is the least severe impairment he is experiencing. Thus, if it were included in the PIP at all, it would not be entered first. Remember that *treatment modality does not inform impairment prioritization in the PIP. Rather, impairment prioritization should inform treatment modality selection.*

Because the Family Dysfunction does seem to center on Eddie's School Avoidance and Tantrums, listing this impairment separately in the PIP is most likely redundant. Remember to avoid "stuffing" the PIP with impairments. Reviewers will no doubt value clinicians whose assessment of patients provides the greatest amount of useful information supplied via the smallest possible amount of data.

Goals and Objectives

Eddie's Treatment Goals and Patient Objectives

Eddie's impairments seem relatively straightforward at this time. Once-weekly family therapy was prescribed as the sole form of treatment because all of his impairments appeared strongly interrelated. Based on the acute nature of his problems and their apparent link to a recent family stressor (mother's surgery), a short-term treatment was proposed. The following are *suggestions* only:

Case Presentation 17: Eddie Patient Impairment Profile		
	Severity rating	
Impairment	**10/15/2001**	**Endpoint goal**
1. Tantrums	2	0
2. School Avoidance	1	0
3. Somatization	1	0

Patient Objectives
To Be Addressed by Treatment Completion: 12/10/2001 **Tantrums** Patient will verbalize • Acceptance of the responsibility for coping with the Tantrums • Awareness of the precipitants of Tantrums • Awareness of the negative consequences of Tantrums • Warning signs that Tantrums are exacerbating • A plan of action to be taken should the Tantrums exacerbate Patient will demonstrate • Participation in the prescribed treatment program • Ability to verbalize, versus act on, anger • Elimination of Tantrums, as evidenced by a normal range score on the Eyberg Child Behavior Inventory • A completed self-care (discharge) plan, including steps to be taken should the Tantrums return or exacerbate *(continued)*

School Avoidance

Patient will verbalize

- Acceptance of the responsibility for coping with School Avoidance
- Awareness of the precipitants of School Avoidance
- Awareness of the negative consequences of School Avoidance
- Warning signs that the School Avoidance is exacerbating
- A plan of action to be taken should the School Avoidance exacerbate

Patient will demonstrate

- Participation in the prescribed treatment program
- Elimination of School Avoidance as evidenced by a normal pattern of regular school attendance
- A completed self-care (discharge) plan, including steps to be taken should the School Avoidance return or exacerbate

Somatization

Patient will verbalize

- Acceptance of the responsibility for coping with Somatization
- Awareness of the precipitants of Somatization
- Warning signs that Somatization is exacerbating
- A plan of action to be taken should the Somatization exacerbate

Patient will demonstrate

- Participation in the prescribed treatment program
- Ability to obtain parental attention with constructive alternative behaviors
- Elimination of Somatization
- A completed self-care (discharge) plan, including steps to be taken should the Somatization return or exacerbate

Goals and Objectives

Goals and Objectives:
Study Questions—Eddie

Instructions: *Read each of the questions below and circle the* most *correct response.*

1. If an impairment receives a severity of 1 or 2, the treatment goal for this impairment

    a) could be any severity rating.
    b) could be any severity rating less than or equal to the original severity rating.
    c) will always be a lower severity rating.
    d) will always be 0.

2. Eddie's projected treatment completion is listed as 12/10/2001. This implies that

    a) treatment will terminate on that date regardless of patient status.
    b) the clinician believes it is reasonable to predict that treatment will be completed by that date.
    c) the reviewer has authorized treatment only until that date.
    d) the clinician is simply setting an arbitrary date for review purposes.

3. If, through the course of treatment, Eddie's Family Dysfunction emerges as a more pervasive problem than originally expected

    a) the clinician must provide behavioral evidence (statements/actions) to support this PIP change.
    b) the clinician can add this impairment to the PIP, with related patient objectives and an additional treatment goal.
    c) both a and b.
    d) none of the above.

4. Eddie's patient objectives for Tantrums include verbalizing "warning signs that Tantrums are exacerbating." This could be evidenced by

    a) Eddie telling his parents, "I am getting mad now" instead of screaming.
    b) Eddie successfully identifying "fist-clenching" as a precursor to Tantrums.
    c) Eddie being aware that his Tantrums are becoming more frequent.
    d) both a and b.

5. Each of Eddie's impairments includes the objective, "participation in the prescribed treatment program." Accomplishing this objective

    a) is contingent on his parents also becoming identified patients.
    b) can theoretically be done without any treatment for Eddie's parents, based on his current PIP.
    c) is contingent on the accuracy of the clinician's original evaluation of Eddie's Family Dysfunction.
    d) both b and c.

6. The treatment goal for Eddie's Somatization is 0. To accomplish this, there *must* be

    a) corroboration of impairment repair by the school nurse.
    b) no further incidence of any headache or stomachache.
    c) no organic expression of psychological disturbances.
    d) both b and c.

Turn the page for the answers to these questions.

Goals and Objectives:
Answers to Study Questions

1. Answer "b" is correct. Obviously, a treatment goal would never involve a greater severity (Answer "a"), which signals increased dysfunction. In chronic cases, however, *maintenance* goals can involve maintaining the current level of severity as opposed to further decompensation. Simply because an impairment receives a severity of 1 or 2 does not guarantee the feasibility of complete (Answer "d") or even partial ("Answer "c") repair.

2. Answer "b" is correct. Projected treatment completion dates are "goals" in themselves and cannot be viewed as absolutes (Answer "a"). As with any other documented changes, modification of this date must be supported with behavioral evidence. The date might also reflect authorization status (Answer "c"), but authorization should always be informed by the clinician's judgment. Furthermore, authorization should never influence the clinician's decision to view treatment as *completed*. A patient who still needs treatment should continue to receive treatment or be transferred to affordable treatment, regardless of authorization.

3. Answer "c" is correct. The clinician can certainly add impairments to the PIP (Answer "b") as treatment progresses. To do so, however, new behavioral evidence must support such additions (Answer "a").

4. Answer "d" is correct. No "correct set" of specific statements or actions is associated with the generic objective "verbalize warning signs that tantrums are exacerbating." Any evidence must, however, be behavioral and as objective as possible. Stating that Eddie is aware of increased Tantrum frequency (Answer "c") constitutes a *conclusion* rather than behavioral evidence.

5. Answer "d" is correct. Even though family therapy might be used as the primary mode of treatment, Eddie's PIP does not include Family Dysfunction *at this time* (Answer "c"). In addition, other treatment modalities (e.g., individual child play therapy, behavior therapy) might be chosen by the clinician, thereby precluding substantial parental involvement (Answer "b"). Furthermore, even with family therapy, treatment would presumably *involve* Eddie's parents but *focus* on Eddie. Finally, regardless of whether Eddie is experiencing a Family Dysfunction, only one identified patient (Eddie) is needed to communicate Eddie's treatment concerns via the PIP (Answer "a").

6. Answer "c" is correct. By definition, treatment goals are accomplished when impairments are totally repaired, and Somatization is defined as "organic expression of psychological disturbances." Corroboration by the school nurse might serve as supportive behavioral evidence (i.e., statements), but only the clinician's judgment is *required* for determining status of treatment goals (Answer "a"). Furthermore, Eddie could certainly continue to report occasional headaches and stomachaches in the future, provided that these symptoms were assessed as legitimate physical problems without psychological roots (Answer "b").

The Treatment Plan

Selecting Interventions

In this chapter, we illustrate how patient goals and objectives can be used as a basis for selecting practitioner interventions. This is illustrated by continuing with the two example cases. Then, an additional new case provides the clinician an opportunity to develop an additional Patient Impairment Profile (PIP), see its links to goals and objectives, and study how intervention choices logically follow from this information.

Definitions

discharge plan   A prescribed course of action to be implemented when the patient is released or dismissed from a treatment setting or treatment, based on an assessment of the patient's status and need for continuing care.

intervention   An action taken by a trained mental health professional to modify, resolve, or stabilize the patient's impairment.

treatment modality   A group or sequence of practitioner interventions used as part of a therapeutic clinical service (e.g., individual psychotherapy).

treatment plan   A patient clinical record that contains the assessment, diagnosis, PIP (including initial and updated severity ratings), patient objectives (with patient progress updates), treatment goals, interventions (initial and current), and discharge plan.

Practitioners select *interventions*, which must be consistent with the patient's goals and objectives. When treatment involves several practitioners, it typically also includes a variety of modalities. Given that the *treatment plan* is the patient's, however, and not the practitioner's, it is useful to organize the plan by *treatment modality* (e.g., individual psychotherapy, group therapy, biofeedback) rather than by practitioner (e.g., psychiatrist, occupational therapist, social worker). It is also important to remember that such a plan must include a *discharge plan.*

Treatment plans, like the PIP, should reflect actual (current) versus potential (future) conditions. Thus, just as potential future impairments should not be cited in the PIP, potential future modalities should not be included in the treatment plan. These can be documented if and when implementation actually occurs.

When using the PIP, it is important to note that specific definitions are given to the terms *treatment plan, goal, objective,* and *intervention.* Much confusion and inconsistency exists regarding these terms, but they must be used uniformly if effective universal communication via the PIP is to be accomplished. Even though these terms have already been defined previously, the following distinctions deserve repeating: First, the treatment plan is the *patient's* treatment plan. Likewise, goals and objectives are also ascribed to the patient. Indeed, only *interventions* are attributed to the clinician. Collectively, these designations reflect that today's managed care environment is less concerned with "how the practitioner is managing the patient" and more with "how the patient is managing."

Selecting Interventions for April's Treatment Plan
(Case 11 continued)

The following patient treatment plan was developed by the treatment team at the inpatient facility where April was admitted. The primary practitioner provided assessment, diagnosis, the initial PIP, and proposed treatment modalities to the team. Then the team members provided further assessment and input to the PIP, as well as individual interventions within the modalities, including discharge planning. Because April recently complained of extrapyramidal side effects from Haldol (haloperidol), her treatment plan included a switch to Risperdal (risperidone). Although Risperdal is more expensive, it was chosen as a cost-effective alternative because it has less acute side effects and causes less long-term risk of tardive dyskinesia.

Remember that, as the patient, April provided the basis for the PIP, objectives, and goals. In light of her PIP, this initial treatment plan is intended to address only April's *interim* goals (i.e., involving discharge from the inpatient unit). The following treatment plan contains *suggestions* only.

The Treatment Plan: Selecting Interventions

Treatment Plan for Case Presentation 11: April

Case Presentation 11: April **Patient Impairment Profile**		
	Severity rating	
Impairment	**4/10/2001**	**Interim goal**
1. Delusions (Nonparanoid)	4	2
2. Psychotic Thought/Behavior	3	2
3. Inadequate Self-Maintenance Skills	2	1
4. Educational Performance Deficit	2	2

Patient Objectives

To Be Addressed by Discharge From Inpatient Setting to Group Home Setting: 4/16/2001

See Chapter 5 for a complete list of April's patient objectives.

Practitioner Interventions

Delusions (Nonparanoid)

Psychopharmacotherapy:
- Assess psychotropic medication status.
- Treat Delusions with Risperdal (risperidone) 1 mg twice daily; increase over 3 days to 3 mg twice daily.

Nursing:
- House patient on locked ward and reduce restrictions as appropriate.
- Continually assess patient's readiness to resume unsupervised activities and move to an unlocked unit.
- Ensure that patient receives medication as prescribed.
- Monitor vital signs and behavior at regular intervals.

Discharge planning services:
- Assess appropriate level of service (e.g., group home versus semi-independent living) for patient upon discharge.
- Obtain living arrangement reservations for patient upon discharge.
- Establish communication network for continuity of care upon discharge.

(continued)

Psychotic Thought/Behavior

Psychopharmacotherapy:
- Assess psychotropic medication status.
- Treat Psychotic Thought/Behavior with Risperdal (risperidone) 1 mg twice daily; increase over 3 days to 3 mg twice daily.

Nursing:
- House patient on locked ward and reduce restrictions as appropriate.
- Continually assess patient's readiness to resume unsupervised activities and move to an unlocked unit.
- Ensure that patient receives medication as prescribed.
- Monitor vital signs and behavior at regular intervals.

Discharge planning services:
- Assess appropriate level of service (e.g., group home versus semi-independent living) for patient upon discharge.
- Obtain living arrangement reservations for patient upon discharge.
- Establish communication network for continuity of care upon discharge.

Inadequate Self-Maintenance Skills

Psychopharmacotherapy:
- Assess extent to which Inadequate Self-Maintenance Skills are secondary to recent decline in antipsychotic medication level.

Nursing:
- Establish behavioral contract, rewarding improved self-maintenance skills with increased privileges (e.g., move to unlocked unit).
- Assess readiness for group therapy.

Discharge planning services:
- Assess appropriate level of service (e.g., group home versus semi-independent living) for patient upon discharge.
- Establish communication network for continuity of care upon discharge.

Educational Performance Deficit

Discharge planning services:
- Schedule patient for psychological testing, unless recently performed, to assess for Learning Disability and general intelligence.
- Suggest that patient be enrolled in remedial program for Educational Performance Deficit upon discharge.

The Treatment Plan: Selecting Interventions

Note that the interventions for both April's Delusions and her Psychotic Thought/Behavior are identical. They are listed here for illustrative purposes. When communicating with a managed care organization, it may be completely feasible to cite identical interventions only once, with reference to two or more impairments. In most cases, however, impairments will be sufficiently unique to warrant separate interventions.

Selecting Interventions for Billy's Treatment Plan
(Case 12 continued)

The clinician to whom Billy was referred decided that treatment would not necessitate any referrals for supplemental services. Thus, this practitioner was solely responsible for the development of Billy's treatment plan. After making the initial assessment of diagnosis, PIP, goals, and objectives, the clinician decided that one treatment modality (family therapy) would suffice. Then individual interventions within this modality were chosen with respect to the impairments in the PIP. As the patient, Billy provided the basis for the PIP, objectives, and goals. Given his straightforward PIP, the initial treatment plan was designed to address Billy's *endpoint goals* (i.e., the repair of his impairments). The following treatment plan contains *suggestions* only.

Treatment Plan for Case Presentation 12: Billy

Case Presentation 12: Billy Patient Impairment Profile		
	Severity rating	
Impairment	7/2/2001	Endpoint goal
1. Enuresis	1	0
2. Pathological Guilt	1	0

Patient Objectives
To Be Addressed by Treatment Completion: 8/13/2001
See Chapter 5 for a complete list of Billy's patient objectives.

Practitioner Interventions

Enuresis

Family therapy:

- Assess for Concomitant Medical Condition (e.g., confirm that recent physical examination results have been unremarkable).
- Assess the appropriateness of suggesting that Billy's grandmother be invited to a treatment session(s).
- Educate Billy and his parents regarding the prevalence and treatability of Enuresis.
- Initiate behavior modification via a nocturnal alarm system, scheduled voiding, restricted nighttime drinking, and the use of a star chart for positive performance tracking and reinforcement.
- Educate Billy's parents regarding the availability of medication as an adjunct treatment (e.g., imipramine, 25–50 mg/day) should behavior modification prove insufficient.

Pathological Guilt

Family therapy:

- Assess extent to which Pathological Guilt is limited to Enuresis.
- Validate Billy's thoughts and feelings regarding his "messing" and his relationships with his parents and grandmother.
- Educate Billy (and his parents and/or grandmother) that wetting the bed is accidental behavior that he can learn to control, not bad behavior that should be punished.
- Initiate role-playing with Billy and his parents to clarify the difference between accidents and intentional wrongdoing.
- Suggest that Billy and his parents establish "house rules" regarding "what to do when you do something wrong" (to facilitate healthy forgiveness behavior and help prevent future Pathological Guilt).

Step 5: Selecting Interventions

One new case follows. As in Chapter 5, you will create an Impairment Inventory (Steps 1 and 2) and then construct a PIP (Step 3). Goals and objectives (Step 4) are listed next, providing a basis for addressing interventions (Step 5). Interventions, like goals and objectives, cannot be reduced to one "correct" set for any given case. Such decisions are made by the clinician in collaboration with the patient. Thus, multiple-choice questions about interventions are presented to facilitate integration of this new information with previous topics (i.e., impairments, severities, the PIP, goals, and objectives). Once again, please read the vignette and imagine that you are actually interviewing the identified patient.

The Treatment Plan: Selecting Interventions

Notes

Turn the page for the next case.

138   Casebook for Managing Managed Care

Case Presentation 18
"Karen"

Reason for Referral

Karen, a 16-year-old Asian American girl, was referred to you by a local crisis center for troubled teens. She has been staying at the center's temporary shelter for the past 4 days after running away from home. Her parents know her whereabouts. Karen reports her reason for running away was that "my parents try to enforce stupid rules, and they treat me like a 4-year-old." You agree to see Karen on the condition that her parents and 11-year-old brother come in as well. You interview the family and obtain the following information:

History

Karen's mother tells you that this is the "third or fourth" time that Karen has run away in the past year and a half. Prior to this occurrence, she was "only gone for a day or two, but this time Karen said she was never coming back." Karen interrupts to say that her mother "makes too big a deal" of these incidents and adds that "I only run away when there is nothing else left to do." Karen objects to her curfew "which none of my friends have." She feels this is especially unfair because "I do okay in school." Karen's mother replies that without the curfew "she would probably be out all night doing who knows what." Her mother also complains that Karen "has started lying all the time, telling even stupid lies that are obviously untrue."

When asked about the origin of these problems, Karen's father shrugs and says, "I never have any real problems with her." Regarding the recent lying, he chuckles, stating, "She can't pull it off with me. I see it in her eyes." Karen's mother seems angered by this comment and proceeds to recount a list of offenses. She cites occasions when Karen has lied (e.g., regarding her whereabouts, whether she completed assignments); refused to do her chores; or slammed her door, locked herself in her room, and "blasted that awful music." She also claims that Karen "has something to say about everything I ask, and I'm sick of her temper and rebelliousness." Karen protests, stating, "I shouldn't have to listen to her. I'm not a little kid anymore!"

Clinical Presentation

Karen presents as a tall, slender adolescent wearing a fashionable sweater, blue jeans, and black boots. She is alert and coherent but also angry and impatient. Her speech is normal, but she raises her voice often, speaking over her mother. Her eye contact is almost glaring, suggesting a defiant attitude. When questioned about the potential dangers of running away, she replies, "I can take care of myself just fine. I'm not dumb."

Karen's father sits quietly next to her through most of the interview, but he also shows signs of impatience (e.g., looking at his watch). He does not seem to believe that there are any significant problems, explaining that "I had to push the limits at her age a bit, too. Besides, I think I might have taken off, too, if my mother had been on me all the time." Karen's mother, seated by her son, is visibly angry and holds back tears on several occasions. She glares at both Karen and her husband as she describes the home situation. Meanwhile, Karen's brother appears bored throughout much of the interview. He primarily stares at the floor, but he does wince occasionally when Karen and her mother begin arguing.

Assessment Assumptions

No sexual, physical, or substance abuse is present. All factors not explicitly mentioned above have been ruled out. In your waiting room, Karen's mother completed the Eyberg Child Behavior Inventory (Burns and Patterson 1990), unassisted by Karen's father who had "no interest in filling out lots of forms." Karen's scores were 3 standard deviations above the mean, suggesting severe behavior problems.

> **DSM-IV Axis I diagnosis**: 313.81 Oppositional defiant disorder
> **DSM-IV Axis II diagnosis**: None

Identify the impairments and rate their severities on the next page.

The Treatment Plan: Selecting Interventions 139

Steps 1 & 2:
Identifying Impairments and Rating Severity

Instructions: *List **all the impairments,** with their respective **severity ratings.** After each, cite **behavioral evidence (statements/actions)** that supports your choices of both impairments and severities. List the impairments that refer **only to Karen.** Remember that information **not** mentioned should be assumed to be **nonapplicable** to this patient (e.g., no organic pathology is present). Assume that all symptoms and/or relevant information are reported in the case description.*

Impairment Inventory	
Impairment	**Severity rating**
1.	
Behavioral evidence:	
2.	
Behavioral evidence:	
3.	
Behavioral evidence:	
4.	
Behavioral evidence:	
5.	
Behavioral evidence:	

Turn the page for Impairment Inventory and severity rating answers.

Impairment Inventory	
(Impairments are listed chronologically as they appear in the vignette.)	
Impairment	**Severity rating**
1. Running Away *(critical)*	**3** *(Severely incapacitating)*
Behavioral evidence: This is the "third or fourth" time Karen has run away in the past year and a half, in each case for a day or two, but this time "Karen said she was never coming back." She shows poor insight regarding the risk of danger, stating, "I can take care of myself just fine." She did, however, go to a shelter for help.	
2. Lying *(noncritical)*	**1** *(Distressing)*
Behavioral evidence: Karen "has started lying all the time, telling even stupid lies that are obviously untrue." Her mother cites recent occasions when Karen has lied (e.g., about where she was going, whether she completed assignments).	
3. Oppositionalism *(noncritical)*	**2** *(Destabilizing)*
Behavioral evidence: Karen has recently lied, refused to do her chores, or locked herself in her room and "blasted that awful music." Her mother reports that Karen also "has something [rebellious] to say about everything I ask." Karen protests, stating, "I shouldn't have to listen to her. I'm not a little kid anymore!" Karen's Eyberg Child Behavior Inventory scores were 3 standard deviations above the mean, suggesting severe behavior problems.	
4. Family Dysfunction *(noncritical)*	**2** *(Destabilizing)*
Behavioral evidence: Karen's father shows little motivation (e.g., looks at his watch). He states, "I never have any real problems with her," explaining that "I had to push the limits at her age a bit too....I think I might have taken off, too, if my mother had been on me all the time." Karen's mother is visibly angry, holds back tears, and glares at both Karen and her husband as she describes the home situation.	

Common Errors

Marital/Relationship Dysfunction: There is clear behavioral support for this impairment regarding *Karen's parents*. With Karen as the identified patient, however, impairments must directly apply to her. Thus, it is more appropriate to cite a Family Dysfunction, which provides a rationale for treating Karen's parents' problems *as they directly relate to the identified patient*. Moreover, Karen's behaviors also contribute directly to the Family Dysfunction.

Tantrums: Karen's defiant yelling might be viewed as a "dramatic outburst," but she is not "crying, kicking, or screaming." Remember that strict adherence to the *specific operational definitions in the Impairment Lexicon* is necessary for reliable communication (e.g., between clinicians and reviewers).

Create the Patient Impairment Profile (PIP) on the next page.

The Treatment Plan: Selecting Interventions   **141**

Step 3: Creating the Patient Impairment Profile

Instructions: *Now, select those impairments from Karen's Impairment Inventory that will be the current focus of treatment. List them with their respective severity ratings on the Patient Impairment Profile below. List the impairments in **prioritized order**. Then, in the space below, write your rationale for your ranking of each. Remember that information **not** mentioned should be assumed to be **nonapplicable** to this patient.*

Patient Impairment Profile	
Impairment	**Severity rating**
1.	
2.	
3.	
4.	

1. Prioritization rationale:

2. Prioritization rationale:

3. Prioritization rationale:

4. Prioritization rationale:

Turn the page for prioritized PIP answers.

Case Presentation 18: Karen **Patient Impairment Profile**	
Impairment	**Severity rating**
1. Running Away	3
2. Oppositionalism	2
3. Family Dysfunction	2
4. Lying	1

1. Prioritization rationale: This severely incapacitating impairment (severity of 3) must be eliminated because it places Karen at significant risk for harm, and it also appears to be escalating (e.g., from being "gone a night or two" to threatening to never return).

2. Prioritization rationale: Karen must acquire more effective coping skills to replace her current coping via oppositional behavior, which is ultimately self-defeating and can serve to worsen stress levels.

3. Prioritization rationale: Karen's parents' relationship with each other and with Karen is problematic. As such, treatment options might include addressing systemic issues to facilitate Karen's progress and to prevent recidivism.

4. Prioritization rationale: The accuracy of Karen's reporting will have a significant effect on any individual and/or family work. Increasing truthfulness will not only indicate the development of good rapport but also will facilitate treatment and enhance adaptive coping skills.

Common Error

Oppositionalism: Some clinicians might want to prioritize this impairment first in the PIP, while viewing Running Away as a problem subsumed by Oppositionalism. Oppositionalism does involve "pervasive disobedience," and Running Away may be conceptualized as simply one type of disobedience. However, Karen's problems include *potentially dangerous* (severity of 3) behaviors, which can be described only by citing a *critical* impairment. Running Away is a critical impairment, but Oppositionalism is not. Thus, Karen's PIP shows that *when a noncritical impairment (e.g., Oppositionalism) is associated with critical behavior, a critical impairment (e.g., Running Away) also must be cited.* Conversely, Oppositionalism also must be cited because Karen's defiant behavior is not limited to Running Away.

The Treatment Plan: Selecting Interventions

Step 4: Identifying Goals and Objectives

Karen's case can be conceptualized in a variety of viable ways, but the practitioner chose to view Karen's individual problems as manifestations of a larger Family Dysfunction. Given the severity of her Running Away, however, with her apparently rebellious stance toward authority figures, the clinician decided that both individual and family therapy should be used. Individual therapy with Karen would initially be aimed at developing rapport and providing Karen with an "ally" within the family system. To accomplish this, the clinician saw Karen both individually and with the family, respectively, on alternate weeks. On weeks when family therapy precluded individual time, Karen was invited to write down her concerns and leave them with the clinician, to be discussed at her next individual session. Because the clinician hoped that outpatient therapy would suffice, the initial goals based on her PIP were also cited as endpoint goals. The following goals and objectives are *suggestions* only:

Treatment Plan for Case Presentation 18: Karen

Case Presentation 18: Karen Patient Impairment Profile		
	Severity rating	
Impairment	1/12/2001	Endpoint goal
1. Running Away	3	0
2. Oppositionalism	2	0
3. Family Dysfunction	2	0
4. Lying	1	0

Patient Objectives

To Be Addressed by Treatment Completion: 3/12/2001
Running Away

Patient will verbalize
- Acceptance of the responsibility for the running-away behavior
- The potential dangers of Running Away
- The adverse consequences of Running Away
- The precipitants of running-away behavior
- Alternative coping responses
- A plan of action to be taken should the urge to run away return

Patient will demonstrate
- Adherence to the prescribed treatment program
- The ability to prevent Running Away by coping with its precipitants
- Elimination of running-away behavior
- A completed self-care (discharge) plan, including steps to be taken should the urge to run away return

(continued)

Oppositionalism

Patient will verbalize

- Acceptance of the responsibility for coping with the Oppositionalism
- Awareness of the precipitants of Oppositionalism
- Awareness of the adverse consequences of Oppositionalism and the value of compliance
- A plan of action to be taken should the Oppositionalism exacerbate

Patient will demonstrate

- Participation in the prescribed treatment program
- The ability to constructively verbalize, rather than act on, anger
- The ability to cope constructively with restrictions imposed by authority figures
- Elimination of Oppositionalism, as evidenced by a normal-range score on the Eyberg Child Behavior Inventory
- A completed self-care (discharge) plan, including steps to be taken should the Oppositionalism return or exacerbate

Family Dysfunction

Patient will verbalize

- Acceptance of the mutual responsibility for coping with the Family Dysfunction
- Understanding of dysfunctional roles in the family
- Awareness of the benefits derived from functional family roles

Patient will demonstrate

- Participation in the prescribed treatment program
- The ability to participate in family discussion and resolution of problems
- The ability to perform an age-appropriate role within the family
- Elimination of the contribution to Family Dysfunction
- A completed self-care (discharge) plan, including steps to be taken should the Family Dysfunction return or exacerbate

Lying

Patient will verbalize

- Admission of, and acceptance of the responsibility for, Lying
- Awareness of the adverse consequences of Lying and the value of honesty
- Awareness of the precipitants of Lying
- Warning signs that the urge to lie is exacerbating
- A plan of action to be taken should the Lying exacerbate

Patient will demonstrate

- Participation in the prescribed treatment program
- The ability to apologize for past lies and replace them with the truth
- The ability to replace Lying with adaptive coping strategies
- Elimination of Lying
- A completed self-care (discharge) plan, including steps to be taken should the Lying return

The Treatment Plan: Selecting Interventions　　　　　　　　　　　　　　　　　145

　　　If the identified patient is a child (versus parent), a Family Dysfunction presents a special challenge when formulating patient objectives. First, this impairment typically cannot be resolved by one person, particularly when that person has no authority (e.g., a child). Second, factors maintaining the Family Dysfunction often can be outside the child's control (e.g., dysfunctional parenting behavior). Thus, objectives signaling the identified patient's progress can refer only to behaviors (statements/actions) within that patient's control.

　　　In such cases, it might be more useful to propose that parents also be identified as separate patients. Then, their patient objectives—with the child's—can *collectively* provide a comprehensive description of the progress needed for repair of the Family Dysfunction. However, whether one or multiple family members are identified patients, all family members can be targeted by the practitioner's interventions (e.g., for the Family Dysfunction). This strategy is described in the continued discussion of Karen's case that follows.

Step 5: Selecting Interventions

Based on the previously discussed assessment, diagnosis, and proposed treatment modalities, the clinician selected the interventions listed below. Remember that, as the patient, Karen provided the basis for the PIP, goals, and objectives. The following interventions, representing the continuation of Karen's treatment plan described previously, are *suggestions* only:

Treatment Plan for Case Presentation 18: Karen
(continued)

Practitioner Interventions

Running Away

Family therapy:
- Validate both Karen's and her mother's respective feelings.
- Assess and/or confront Karen's father's apparent lack of concern.
- Encourage Karen's parents to develop a mutually agreed on behavioral contract—in session—regarding Karen's Running Away.

Individual therapy:
- Assess Karen's level of insight regarding the potential danger involved in her Running Away.
- Encourage Karen to identify the goals of her Running Away (e.g., alleviation of frustration, communication of dissatisfaction).
- Suggest alternative, adaptive coping responses to Karen.

(continued)

Oppositionalism

Family therapy:

- Assess ways in which oppositional behavior functions within the family system (e.g., effects on parent-child and parent-parent dyads).
- Encourage Karen's parents to develop a mutually agreed on behavioral contract—in session—regarding Karen's Oppositionalism.

Individual therapy:

- Validate Karen's apparent experience of low frustration tolerance.
- Confront Karen regarding the negative consequences of Oppositionalism.
- Encourage Karen to identify the goals of her Oppositionalism (e.g., alleviation of frustration, communication of dissatisfaction).
- Suggest alternative, adaptive coping responses to Karen.
- Reinforce (via verbal praise) Karen's attempts at adaptive coping.

Family Dysfunction

Family therapy:

- Assess the necessity/benefit of including Karen's brother in sessions.
- Assess Karen's parents' apparent Marital/Relationship Dysfunction.
- Encourage Karen's parents to develop mutually agreed on "house rules"—in session—regarding privileges, limits, and responsibilities for both children.
- Support Karen's parents' efforts to improve their relationship and their ability to function as a parenting "team."

Lying

Family therapy:

- Encourage Karen's parents to develop a mutually agreed on behavioral contract—in session—regarding Karen's Lying.

Individual therapy:

- Encourage Karen to identify the goals of her Lying.
- Suggest alternative, adaptive coping responses to Karen.
- Reinforce (via verbal praise) Karen's attempts at adaptive coping.

Note that each impairment need not be addressed by each treatment modality (e.g., Karen's Family Dysfunction). Conversely, intervention lists can at times appear somewhat redundant (e.g., encouraging Karen's parents to develop a behavioral contract). This enables the clinician to communicate that the *same* intervention will be used to treat *more than one* impairment. In Karen's case, the clinician planned to help the parents develop *one* behavioral contract, which would include stipulations for Running Away, Oppositionalism, and Lying.

The Treatment Plan: Selecting Interventions

Practitioner Interventions:
Study Questions—Karen

Instructions: *Read each of the questions below and circle the* most *correct response.*

1. According to the PIP system, the development of therapeutic rapport or alliance between the clinician and Karen could be classified as

    a) a goal.
    b) an objective.
    c) an intervention.
    d) none of the above.

2. Incorporating an intervention in the identified patient's treatment plan that primarily targets someone *other* than the identified patient (e.g., a family member) is acceptable

    a) never, according to the PIP system.
    b) if that other individual also needs treatment.
    c) if doing so is expected to have a direct effect on the identified patient's impairment(s).
    d) when interventions targeting the identified patient are not effective.

3. Selected interventions in the treatment plan should be documented as changed, added, or deleted

    a) whenever the clinician wants to do so.
    b) only when the clinician *actually implements* such modifications.
    c) in response to intervention efficacy and/or patient progress.
    d) b and c.

4. The practitioner should document potential future interventions in the patient treatment plan

    a) never, according to the PIP system.
    b) when such interventions are anticipated as the next phase of treatment.
    c) to communicate long-term plans to the case reviewer.
    d) as a backup resource, when initial interventions are seen as having a low probability of success.

5. According to the PIP system, "utilization of a behavioral contract" could be classified as

    a) a goal.
    b) an objective.
    c) an intervention.
    d) none of the above.

Turn the page for the answers to these questions.

Practitioner Interventions: Answers to Study Questions

1. Answer "b" is correct. Developing therapeutic rapport can never be a goal (Answer "a") because such an alliance is only a precursor to productive treatment participation. It cannot be an intervention (Answer "c") because it is not merely an action performed by the clinician. Although the clinician has a primary responsibility to *facilitate* the patient's attempts to engage in treatment—and is involved in the relational process of building rapport—the development of such a therapeutic alliance completely depends on the patient. Thus, developing such an alliance can be seen as a preliminary objective, signaling patient progress toward whatever treatment goals have been identified in the PIP.

2. Answer "c" is correct. Interventions are "action[s] taken...to modify, resolve, or stabilize the patient's impairment." Such actions can thus target persons other than the patient, provided that they "modify, resolve, or stabilize the patient's impairment." Moreover, such interventions need not be cited only as a last resort (Answer "d") but can be initial treatment strategies. For example, "support[ing] Karen's parents' efforts to improve their relationship and their ability to function as a parenting team" is cited as an initial intervention because it is expected to directly affect Karen's Family Dysfunction. In contrast, interventions on an identified patient's PIP cannot target another person simply because that person needs treatment (Answer "b"). Rather, the other person's independent needs for treatment merit documentation on a separate PIP.

3. Answer "d" is correct. Modifying intervention lists is not done purely at the clinician's discretion (Answer "a"). Rather, such modifications reflect the actual course of treatment (Answer "c") and represent one of the dynamic components of the patient treatment plan. In addition, cited interventions cannot reflect anticipated changes or progress but must only depict currently used strategies (Answer "b"). A history of all interventions used over the entire course of treatment does not belong in the treatment plan. Such information can appropriately be included, however, in the discharge/termination summary.

4. Answer "a" is correct. As stated in the answer to Question 3, cited interventions must not depict anticipated treatment methods (Answer "b"), and backup interventions are simply one type of "potential" intervention (Answer "d"). Furthermore, the patient treatment plan never reflects the *assumption* that treatment will involve long-term care (Answer "c"). Rather, the goal of the briefest possible effective treatment is always implicit, with the assumption that ongoing treatment needs may change over time. In this way, the patient treatment plan—including the PIP—communicates not only why the patient needs treatment *now* but also what treatment is being administered *now*.

5. Answer "b" is correct. "Utilizing a behavioral contract" might be seen as a clinician's intervention, particularly if the clinician suggests it, initiates its development, and continually tracks its success (Answer "c"). As in the answer to Question 1, however, the clinician has only a facilitating role with such a contract. The patient must successfully utilize the behavioral contract to constructively modify maladaptive behavior. Doing so would not constitute a treatment goal, however (Answer "a"). Rather, successful use of such a contract could indicate progress toward a goal (e.g., repair of Oppositionalism) and thus be a valid objective.

Tracking Patient Progress

In this chapter, we show how Patient Impairment Profile (PIP)–based treatment plans can readily portray the current status and progress of ongoing patient care. Once again, the two example cases are used as illustrations. Then an additional new case is presented, permitting the clinician to integrate the PIP, goals, objectives, and interventions with documentation of progress.

Definitions

performance measure A standard or indicator that captures and quantifies the performance of processes and the results or outcomes of care.

process of care A goal-directed, interrelated series of steps, actions, or mechanisms in the rendering of care.

150   **Casebook for Managing Managed Care**

Treatment plans are not static but rather depict the ongoing *process of care*. To maximize the likelihood of treatment authorization, practitioners must regularly communicate a clinical rationale that shows both patient progress and the continued clinical necessity of treatment, which can be done by documenting relevant patient statements or actions. As stated in Chapter 5, providing quantifiable information (e.g., standardized *performance measures)* also can be helpful, particularly when changes are small. In the absence of standardized measures, providing subjectively based numerical data (e.g., "50% improvement") can facilitate communication of progress.

Updating a PIP-based treatment plan involves reassessing each impairment and its severity rating, as well as reevaluating the patient's progress toward meeting the identified goals and objectives.

Tracking April's Progress (Case 11 continued)

Because April had complained of extrapyramidal side effects when receiving Haldol (haloperidol), her medication was switched to Risperdal (risperidone) (as outlined in her treatment plan in Chapter 6). By the third day on the locked unit, her Delusions were markedly reduced, her Psychotic Thought/Behavior had subsided appreciably, and she began to show some awareness that her thoughts and behaviors were abnormal. She reported, "I know I've been acting crazy, but I am feeling all better now with more medicine." She also began asking to return to her semi-independent apartment. In addition, on her third morning on the unit, she asked if she might be able to participate in group activities "because I am bored and I'm sick of just watching TV." Her social behavior was observed as increasingly appropriate.

The treatment team met on the third day to review April's progress. Everyone agreed that she had improved measurably. They suggested that her onset of Inadequate Self-Maintenance Skills had most likely been the result of her recently lowered dosage of antipsychotic medication. Still, she expressed little insight regarding her Delusions and the need to identify warning signs of their reoccurrence. She also continued frequently demonstrating some marked Psychotic Thought/Behavior (e.g., occasional bizarre hand movements, frequent inappropriate laughter, occasional incoherent speech) and some residual Inadequate Self-Maintenance Skills (e.g., occasionally interrupting group activities she had not been asked to join). In addition, the team had not yet addressed her Educational Performance Deficit, given its chronic nature and the more pressing needs concerning her other impairments.

Given April's progress, the team agreed that she should be moved to an unlocked unit, with the condition that she report to the nursing station on an hourly basis. She was scheduled for daily group therapy, with the understanding that making two or more inappropriate interruptions in any group session would result in her being asked to leave for that day. She was also scheduled for various activities through occupational therapy services. Finally, April would report to the nurses' station 5 minutes early for each scheduled medication dose, an intervention aimed at facilitating her transition back to the group home. April signed a treatment contract readily, stating that "I want to get back to my apartment."

Based on this information, April's PIP-based treatment plan was updated as follows:

Tracking Patient Progress

Treatment Plan for Case Presentation 11: April

Case Presentation 11: April
Patient Impairment Profile

Impairment	Severity rating		
	4/10/2001	4/12/2001	Interim goal
1. Delusions (Nonparanoid)	4	2	2
2. Psychotic Thought/Behavior	3	3	2
3. Inadequate Self-Maintenance Skills	2	1	1
4. Educational Performance Deficit	2	2	2

Patient Objectives: Progress Update

To Be Addressed by Discharge From Inpatient Setting to Group Home Setting: 4/16/2001

(*Target Objective—to be met 100%) (% = percent progress)*

Delusions (Nonparanoid)

Patient will verbalize
- Awareness of the presence of delusional thinking **(75%)**
- Acceptance of the responsibility for coping with the Delusions **(25%)**
- Precipitants for the delusional thinking **(25%)**
- Warning signs that the Delusions are exacerbating **(0%)**
- * A plan of action to be taken should the Delusions exacerbate **(0%)**

Patient will demonstrate
- * Absence of Delusions for 72 hours **(50%)**
- Adherence to a prescribed treatment program **(100%)**
- * A completed self-care (discharge) plan, including steps to be taken should the Delusions return or exacerbate **(0%)**

Psychotic Thought/Behavior

Patient will verbalize
- Awareness of the presence of Psychotic Thought/Behavior **(75%)**
- Acceptance of the responsibility for coping with the Psychotic Thought/Behavior **(50%)**
- Precipitants for the Psychotic Thought/Behavior **(50%)**
- Warning signs that the Psychotic Thought/Behavior is exacerbating **(0%)**
- * A plan of action to be taken should the Psychotic Thought/Behavior exacerbate **(0%)**

(continued)

Patient will demonstrate
  * Absence of Psychotic Thought/Behavior for 72 hours **(25%)**
  • Adherence to prescribed treatment program **(100%)**
  * A completed self-care (discharge) plan, including steps to be taken should the Psychotic Thought/Behavior return or exacerbate **(0%)**

To Be Addressed by Completion of Treatment and Resumption of Semi-Independent Living: 6/18/2001

Delusions (Nonparanoid)

Patient will verbalize
  • Awareness that Delusions can resume without maintained adherence to a discharge plan **(0%)**

Patient will demonstrate
  • Maintained adherence to a self-care plan with maintained absence of Delusions **(0%)**

Psychotic Thought/Behavior

Patient will verbalize
  • Awareness that Psychotic Thought/Behavior can resume without maintained adherence to a discharge plan **(0%)**

Patient will demonstrate
  • Maintained adherence to a self-care plan with adequate management of Psychotic Thought/ Behavior **(0%)**

Inadequate Self-Maintenance Skills

Patient will verbalize
  • Awareness of the presence of Inadequate Self-Maintenance Skills **(25%)**
  • Acceptance of the responsibility for coping with the Inadequate Self-Maintenance Skills **(25%)**
  • Awareness of the dangers or adverse consequences of Inadequate Self-Maintenance Skills **(25%)**
  • A plan of action to be taken should the Inadequate Self-Maintenance Skills exacerbate **(0%)**

Patient will demonstrate
  • Adherence to a prescribed treatment program **(100%)**
  • Adequate management of the Inadequate Self-Maintenance Skills **(25%)**
  • A completed self-care (discharge) plan, including steps to be taken should the Inadequate Self-Maintenance Skills return or exacerbate **(0%)**

(continued)

Tracking Patient Progress   153

Educational Performance Deficit

Patient will verbalize
- Awareness of the Educational Performance Deficit and its negative effect **(0%)**
- Acceptance of the responsibility for coping with the Educational Performance Deficit **(0%)**
- Willingness to participate in an Educational Performance Deficit assessment and remediation program **(0%)**

Patient will demonstrate
- Participation in a remediation program **(0%)**

Practitioner Interventions

See Chapter 6 for a complete list of the practitioner's interventions.

The viability and necessity of continued treatment at the current level of care are supported by April's updated treatment plan. It shows that she still requires treatment, but she is making measurable progress. Specifically, this is evident from her severity rating updates (with reference to her interim goals) and from her progress on target objectives. Remember that a *target* objective is an anticipated patient statement or behavior that signals "discharge" to less service-intensive treatment. Currently, April still needs to show additional improvement regarding most of her target objectives. Demonstrable progress has been made, however, in connection with Delusions, Psychotic Thought/Behavior, and her Inadequate Self-Maintenance Skills. No progress has been noted for her Educational Performance Deficit, but the interventions regarding this impairment all pertain to discharge planning services (see Chapter 8). In addition, none of her objectives concerning this impairment are *target* objectives.

Tracking Billy's Progress (Case 12 continued)

During the intake, Billy's parents reported that Billy had no Concomitant Medical Conditions, "and he just had a checkup." The parents were also questioned about Billy's grandmother, and it was decided that it might be helpful for her to "join the team." She was thus invited to attend the next session. The practitioner educated Billy and his parents about Enuresis, emphasizing that it is typically very treatable. Billy responded positively when assured that his parents and the practitioner would "help me stop my problem." Billy's parents agreed to purchase a nocturnal bed-wetting alarm, which they were instructed to bring to the next session. The practitioner also helped them develop a schedule for Billy's nighttime drinking and voiding before bed. Billy also appeared eager to use a star chart to track his performance.

During the second session, the family reviewed the use of the alarm together. Billy responded well to the practitioner's framing this device as a "pretty special machine for a pretty special boy." Because Billy's grandmother also attended this session, the practitioner was able to facilitate the family's processing of "what had happened at Grandma's house." Billy's father asked his mother if she might have been "a bit stern" with Billy, and she acknowledged that this was true. She, in turn, was able to express her frustration that Billy's parents "gave me no idea of Billy's problem, so it took me off guard." The entire family then engaged in role-playing regarding apologies and forgiveness. This exercise seemed particularly helpful to Billy, who was very willing to forgive his grandmother "for scolding." Billy's grandmother also spontaneously suggested that Billy "can also practice with his alarm at my house."

By the third session, Billy was reportedly complying with his treatment, and he had wet his bed only once during the week. Billy enthusiastically presented his star chart to the practitioner, complete with its six out of seven stars. He also appeared quite proud to report that "the alarm woke me up, and I didn't wet the whole bed." During this session, Billy's parents were encouraged to work on developing some "house rules" regarding "what to do when you do something wrong." This included discussing the difference between "doing bad things" and "accidents." Billy was also able to verbalize that "if Mommy and Daddy forgive me, I can feel good and I get another chance!" Billy's mother remarked that Billy seemed to be acting "more and more like a big boy," and this visibly encouraged Billy.

Based on this information, Billy's PIP-based treatment plan was updated as follows:

Treatment Plan for Case Presentation 12: Billy

Case Presentation 12: Billy Patient Impairment Profile			
	Severity rating		
Impairment	7/2/2001	7/16/2001	Endpoint goal
1. Enuresis	1	1	0
2. Pathological Guilt	1	1	0

Patient Objectives: Progress Update

To Be Addressed by Treatment Completion: 8/13/2001
Enuresis
 	
(% = percent progress)
 	
Patient will verbalize
    • Awareness of the presence of Enuresis **(100%)**
    • Acceptance of the responsibility for coping with the Enuresis **(100%)**
    • Willingness to participate in the treatment of Enuresis **(100%)**
    • A plan of action to be taken should the Enuresis exacerbate **(25%)**
Patient will demonstrate
    • Adherence to a prescribed treatment program **(100%)**
    • Elimination of Enuresis **(50%)**
    • A completed self-care (discharge) plan, including steps to be taken should the Enuresis exacerbate **(0%)**
 	
(continued)

Tracking Patient Progress 155

Pathological Guilt

Patient will verbalize
- Awareness of the Pathological Guilt and its current adverse consequences (e.g., generalized anxiety) **(75%)**
- Willingness to participate in the treatment of Pathological Guilt **(100%)**

Patient will demonstrate
- Elimination of Pathological Guilt as evidenced by cessation of repetitive apologizing behavior **(75%)**
- A completed self-care (discharge) plan, including steps to be taken should the Pathological Guilt exacerbate **(0%)**

Practitioner Interventions

See Chapter 6 for a complete list of the practitioner's interventions.

Billy's updated treatment plan also supports the viability and necessity of continued treatment at the current level of care. It shows that he is making good progress but has not yet accomplished all patient objectives or goals. Note that no target objectives are identified because all of Billy's goals are *endpoint* goals, and he is already receiving treatment at a minimally structured level of care (i.e., outpatient family therapy). Thus, accomplishing all goals will simply signal the completion of treatment.

Step 6: Tracking Progress

One new case follows. As in Chapter 6, you will create an Impairment Inventory (Steps 1 and 2) and then construct a PIP (Step 3). Goals and objectives (Step 4) are listed next, followed by interventions (Step 5). Then, progress toward goals and objectives (Step 6) is documented. Based on this hypothetical progress, multiple-choice questions are then presented to facilitate integration of this new information with previous topics (i.e., impairments, severities, the PIP, goals, objectives, and interventions). Once again, please read the vignette and imagine that you are actually interviewing the identified patient.

156   **Casebook for Managing Managed Care**

Case Presentation 19
"Inez"

Reason for Referral

Inez, a 37-year-old Latina woman, and her husband, Joe, a 40-year-old Latino man, have come to see you after Joe called your office. On the telephone, Joe explained that his wife refuses to go outside the house unless he accompanies her because "she's picked up this terrible fear of dogs." She also has been "sleeping in quite a bit, and she used to get up with me. She won't answer the phone or spend time with friends that stop by to visit either." You interview Inez and her husband and obtain the following information:

History

Inez and Joe have been married for 12 years and have no children. Inez is a housewife and reportedly has "always been a bit of an introvert." Still, in the past she has typically maintained four or five friendships with women in her neighborhood with whom she would go shopping, walking, dining, and so forth. Joe is a successful businessman who is active in several civic organizations but "devoted to always making Inez my first priority." They both report a high level of satisfaction with their marriage and "really enjoy doing things together."

When you ask Inez about her fear of dogs, she tells you that she has never been fond of dogs and remembers "being scared of them as a small child." Then, about 6 months ago while walking at a local park, she saw "a large mean-looking dog bite a young girl on the arm." Inez "immediately broke into a cold sweat. My heart started racing, and I felt like running away as fast as I could. I avoided the park after that." She further reports, "I know it seems crazy, but from that point on I just couldn't seem to keep my fear of dogs from growing. I don't really have any other fears—like heights or elevators—like I know some people do. But when it comes to dogs, forget it. Since that day in the park, I don't want to get anywhere near one!" Inez "feels fine" when with her husband, stating, "I can go anywhere with him." Alone, however, she feels completely safe only at home.

Over time, the number of places that Inez avoided (because of her fear of another dog attack) grew until she hardly ever left the house. Soon after, she stopped returning friends' telephone calls and would tell them "I don't feel up to talking now" when they would stop by. She explains, "I'm concerned they will ask me to go out with them and that when I decline, I'll have to explain the real reason that I don't want to go anywhere.

Clinical Presentation

Inez presents as a tall, thin, and casually dressed woman. Joe is also tall, thin, and well groomed. For most of the session, he has a worried expression on his face. Inez appears calm but somewhat sad (e.g., her eyes are typically downcast). When asked how she feels about her current situation, she shrugs and says, "Just awful. I'm afraid to go anywhere without Joe, and when I think of all the things I'm missing out on, it's pretty depressing." When asked about any recurrence of her physical symptoms (e.g., racing heart, cold sweat), she states, "I'm fine unless I see or hear a dog. I know it's silly, but lately it even bothers me to see one on TV. I get scared all over again. I'm starting to wonder if I'll ever get over this." Inez reports that "my husband has been a great support through all this. I can tell him how I am feeling any time, and he always listens." Joe reports that Inez has "done a great job keeping the house up in spite of all this" and that he is willing to "do whatever it takes" to help his wife.

Assessment Assumptions

No hallucinations, delusions, or substance abuse is present. All factors not explicitly mentioned above have been ruled out. In your waiting room, Inez completed the State-Trait Anxiety Inventory for Adults (Spielberger 1983). Her state score (while thinking about dogs) was 2 standard deviations above the mean, reflecting marked symptomatology. Her trait score (in general) was less than 1 standard deviation above the mean, reflecting normative functioning.

> **DSM-IV Axis I diagnosis:** 300.29 Specific phobia
> **DSM-IV Axis II diagnosis:** None

Identify the impairments and rate their severities on the next page.

Tracking Patient Progress 157

Steps 1 & 2:
Identifying Impairments and Rating Severity

Instructions: *List **all the impairments,** with their respective **severity ratings.** After each, cite **behavioral evidence (statements/actions)** that supports your choices of both impairments and severities. List the impairments that refer **only to Inez.** Remember that information **not** mentioned should be assumed to be **nonapplicable** to this patient (e.g., no organic pathology is present). Assume that all symptoms and/or relevant information are reported in the case description.*

Impairment Inventory	
Impairment	**Severity rating**
1.	
Behavioral evidence:	
2.	
Behavioral evidence:	
3.	
Behavioral evidence:	
4.	
Behavioral evidence:	
5.	
Behavioral evidence:	

Turn the page for Impairment Inventory and severity rating answers.

Impairment Inventory	
Impairment	**Severity rating**
1. Phobia *(critical)*	**2** *(Destabilizing)*
Behavioral evidence: Inez refuses to go outside the house unless her husband is with her because "when it comes to dogs, forget it. Since that day in the park, I don't want to get anywhere near one!" On the State-Trait Anxiety Inventory for Adults, her state score (while thinking about dogs) was 2 standard deviations above the mean, reflecting marked symptomatology. Her trait score (in general) was less than 1 standard deviation above the mean, reflecting normative functioning.	
2. Social Withdrawal *(noncritical)*	**2** *(Destabilizing)*
Behavioral evidence: Inez does not return friends' telephone calls and also tells friends she "doesn't feel up to it" when they stop by so that she can avoid going somewhere with them. However, she can "go anywhere" with her husband.	
3. Dysphoric Mood *(critical)*	**2** *(Destabilizing)*
Behavioral evidence: Inez has been "sleeping in quite a bit." She appears sad (e.g., eyes frequently downcast) and says that she feels "just awful" and that "it's pretty depressing" when she thinks about things she is missing out on.	

Common Errors

Anxiety: Inez apparently does experience "a state of uneasiness, worry, apprehension, or dread without sufficient objective justification," but it is entirely limited to her response to dogs. She "feels fine" when with her husband, stating, "I can go anywhere with him." Alone, she feels completely safe at home, and she further reports, "I'm fine unless I see or hear a dog." Inez's case illustrates why the Impairment Lexicon distinguishes between a Phobia and Anxiety. Moreover, her State-Trait Anxiety Inventory for Adults trait score was less than 1 standard deviation above the mean, reflecting normative functioning.

Obsessions: Although Inez does experience "unwelcome...emotions," they occur only in the presence of dogs, in connection with her Phobia. Although it now "even bothers [her] to see one on TV," these emotions do not occur in the absence of her Phobia. In contrast, Obsessions involve "ideas, emotions, or urges that repetitiously...force themselves into consciousness" *independent* of any physical stimulus.

Create the Patient Impairment Profile (PIP) on the next page.

Tracking Patient Progress   **159**

Step 3: Creating the Patient Impairment Profile

Instructions: *Now, select those impairments from Inez's Impairment Inventory that will be the current focus of treatment. List them with their respective severity ratings on the Patient Impairment Profile below. List the impairments in **prioritized order.** Then, in the space below, write your rationale for your ranking of each. Remember that information **not** mentioned should be assumed to be **nonapplicable** to this patient.*

Patient Impairment Profile	
Impairment	**Severity rating**
1.	
2.	
3.	
4.	

1. Prioritization rationale:

2. Prioritization rationale:

3. Prioritization rationale:

4. Prioritization rationale:

Turn the page for prioritized PIP answers.

Case Presentation 19: Inez	
Patient Impairment Profile	
Impairment	**Severity rating**
1. Phobia	2
2. Dysphoric Mood	2
3. Social Withdrawal	2

1. Prioritization rationale: Inez's mood will not improve and she will not be able to spend time with friends until this destabilizing impairment (severity of 2) is treated.

2. Prioritization rationale: Inez has been sleeping in mornings, reports feeling "just awful" about her phobia, and admits that her situation is "pretty depressing." It is very important to work toward resolving this destabilizing (severity of 2) impairment so that she does not become hopeless or despondent.

3. Prioritization rationale: As Inez's phobia is resolved, encouraging her to reconnect with friends and reestablish relationships most likely will help her improve her mood. Resolving this destabilizing (severity of 2) impairment is a tertiary treatment concern.

Common Error

Dysphoric Mood: Because Dysphoric Mood can be considered a more *pervasive* problem and Phobia a more *restricted* problem, some clinicians might want to prioritize Dysphoric Mood first in the PIP. This decision would be supported by the fact that Inez's Dysphoric Mood is one of her most severe (severity of 2) impairments. Remember, however, that *prioritization choices are not based solely on severity ratings.* This becomes obvious when two impairments have the same severity rating. In such cases, it becomes even more crucial that the practitioner have a logical clinical rationale for prioritization. One useful approach to such decisions involves considering if impairment *A* can be expected to improve or worsen *without treatment* of impairment *B* and vice versa. For example, Inez reports that she "feels just awful" (i.e., Dysphoric Mood) specifically *about her Phobia* and related sequelae. Thus, treating her Phobia should help to alleviate her Dysphoric Mood. In contrast, attempting to treat her Dysphoric Mood without addressing her Phobia would probably be ineffective and/or worsen her mood.

Tracking Patient Progress

Step 4: Identifying Goals and Objectives

Because of the apparently circumscribed nature of Inez's impairments, the practitioner viewed Inez as the identified patient in an individual case. Given Inez's extensive dependence on her husband and his great concern for her, however, the practitioner also invited Inez's husband to attend the weekly individual psychotherapy sessions. Short-term outpatient treatment was viewed as sufficient, and initial goals based on her PIP also were cited as endpoint goals. The following goals and objectives are *suggestions* only:

Treatment Plan for Case Presentation 19: Inez

Case Presentation 19: Inez **Patient Impairment Profile**		
	Severity rating	
Impairment	**9/28/2001**	**Endpoint goal**
1. Phobia	2	0
2. Dysphoric Mood	2	0
3. Social Withdrawal	2	0

Patient Objectives
To Be Addressed by Treatment Completion: 11/23/2001 **Phobia** Patient will verbalize<ul><li>Acceptance of the responsibility for coping with the Phobia</li><li>Awareness of the potential links (via conditioned learning) between the Phobia and past (recent and/or remote) experience</li><li>Coping response alternatives to Phobic avoidance</li><li>A plan of action to be taken should the Phobia exacerbate</li></ul> Patient will demonstrate<ul><li>Participation in the prescribed treatment program</li><li>Successful use of relaxation techniques in the presence of the feared stimuli (e.g., dogs shown on television, dogs in the park)</li><li>Ability to pet dogs known to be friendly</li><li>Elimination of the Phobia as evidenced by a normal-range score on the State-Trait Anxiety Inventory for Adults state scale while patient thinks about dogs</li><li>A completed self-care (discharge) plan, including steps to be taken should the Phobia return</li></ul> *(continued)*

Dysphoric Mood

Patient will verbalize
- Acceptance of the responsibility for coping with the Dysphoric Mood
- Statements about self that are realistically positive and hopeful rather than unrealistically negative
- Warning signs that the Dysphoric Mood is exacerbating
- A plan of action to be taken should the Dysphoric Mood exacerbate

Patient will demonstrate
- Adherence to the prescribed treatment program
- Increased self-initiated and self-directed activities
- Elimination of Dysphoric Mood
- A completed self-care (discharge) plan, including steps to be taken should the Dysphoric Mood return or exacerbate

Social Withdrawal

Patient will verbalize
- Acceptance of the responsibility for coping with Social Withdrawal
- Awareness that Social Withdrawal can increase the severity of both Phobia and Dysphoric Mood
- Warning signs that the Social Withdrawal is exacerbating
- A plan of action to be taken should the Social Withdrawal worsen

Patient will demonstrate
- Participation in the prescribed treatment program
- Plans and activities to be initiated with husband or friends at previous (i.e., before impairment onset) frequency levels
- Elimination of Social Withdrawal
- A completed self-care (discharge) plan, including steps to be taken should the Social Withdrawal return or exacerbate

Note that positive behaviors not present *before* impairment onset can still be identified as patient objectives if the clinician assesses these behaviors to be valid indicators of progress toward impairment resolution. For example, demonstrating the "ability to pet dogs known to be friendly" is identified as an objective for Inez, even though she has never been fond of dogs. Because persons without dog Phobia pet dogs with no difficulty, this behavior is a valid objective. Furthermore, it represents a potentially *preventive* step toward ensuring that Inez's Phobia does not recur.

Tracking Patient Progress   **163**

Step 5: Selecting Interventions

Based on the previously discussed assessment, diagnosis, and proposed treatment modalities, the practitioner chose the interventions listed below. Inez's husband did agree to attend her individual therapy sessions. Remember, however, that—as the patient—Inez provided the basis for the PIP, objectives, and goals. The following interventions, representing the continuation of Inez's treatment plan described above, are *suggestions* only:

Treatment Plan for Case Presentation 19: Inez
(continued)

Practitioner Interventions

Phobia

Individual therapy:
- Assess appropriateness of evaluation for antianxiety medication.
- Validate Inez's thoughts and feelings about her Phobia.
- Educate Inez about the potential links between conditioned learning and her Phobia.
- Encourage Inez to explore connections between her Phobia, her childhood fear of dogs, and any relevant childhood experiences.
- Initiate relaxation training and graduated in vivo exposure exercises.

Dysphoric Mood

Individual therapy:
- Assess the extent to which Inez's Dysphoric Mood is independent of her Phobia versus contingent on it.
- Validate her thoughts and feelings about her Dysphoric Mood.
- Suggest that Inez identify all positive facets of her life that are not deleteriously affected by her Phobia.
- Clarify the nature of Inez's apparent shame regarding her Phobia, with respect to disclosing it to friends.
- Encourage Inez to disclose her Phobia to her close friends and to request their emotional support.

Social Withdrawal

Individual therapy:
- Validate Inez's thoughts and feelings about her desire to withdraw.
- Educate her about the exacerbating effects of Social Withdrawal on her other impairments.
- Encourage her to ask one or two friends to resume social activity with her, first with her husband and later without him.

Note that some interventions may seem equally appropriate for two or more impairments (e.g., encouraging Inez to disclose her Phobia might be applied either to Dysphoric Mood or to Social Withdrawal). Because prioritized impairments can still be treated simultaneously, however, matching interventions with impairments is less crucial than choosing appropriate interventions overall for a given patient.

Step 6: Tracking Progress

During the intake, Inez reported that she did not want to "take any drugs if at all possible." The clinician informed her that nonpharmaceutical treatments were available and that her need for antianxiety and/or antidepressant medication would be monitored pending her progress without it. Much of this first session focused on validating Inez's thoughts and feelings about her impairments and on educating her (and her husband) about the potential link between her Phobia and conditioned learning. With this in mind, Inez seemed to be quite encouraged by the notion that a learned Phobia might also be "unlearned." She expressed enthusiastic willingness to begin relaxation training and gradual in vivo exposure exercises. Finally, the practitioner educated her about the exacerbating effects of Social Withdrawal on her other impairments and encouraged her to begin considering how she might address this behavior.

In the second session, the practitioner initiated relaxation training, simultaneously taping this exercise so that Inez could practice it daily at home with the tape. Inez also was instructed to write down as many positive aspects of her life that were still present that she could identify. She was asked to bring this list to the next session. Finally, the practitioner also suggested that Inez and her husband schedule at least one brief outing (e.g., a 15-minute walk) per day.

Inez came to the third session, encouraged that "there are still quite a few positives in my life." In contrast, she reported only limited success with her relaxation tape, stating, "I just can't get over the feeling that this is beyond my control. I feel so stupid." In response, the practitioner facilitated Inez's attempts to clarify her apparent shame response to her Phobia and its concomitant link to her Social Withdrawal. As a result, Inez was able to recall that when she was a child, her father once had scolded her harshly for "being a baby" when she refused to pet a neighbor's large dog. The practitioner offered that this event might have reflected Inez's father's own issues rather than a shortcoming in herself. In addition, her husband told her that he felt she had "nothing to be ashamed of." Inez reported that this was "very helpful." As "homework," the practitioner suggested that Inez disclose her Phobia to her close friends and try gradually to resume socializing with them.

During the fourth session, Inez reported some improvement with her relaxation training. She also was able to stay in the room "when there was a dog on television," but she "couldn't relax at all" during this time. The practitioner encouraged her to note her progress, given that previously she would have left the room or changed the channel. Her husband then reminded her that she was able to relax quite quickly afterward. The practitioner began in vivo exercises during this session, whereby Inez was instructed to relax and then view a videotape of friendly dogs for 30-second intervals. She was able to do this, so as homework she was asked to view this tape daily for increasingly longer intervals. Inez felt this would be easier "now that I am no longer worried about my friends." Specifically, she reported successfully telling each of them during the week about her Phobia, and they were all very supportive. She had also gone out with several of them twice during the week. She was glad to note that "I feel as safe with them as I do with Joe. Then again, I haven't met up with any dogs yet, and I'm not sure I'm ready."

Based on this information, Inez's PIP-based treatment plan was updated as follows:

Tracking Patient Progress   **165**

Treatment Plan for Case Presentation 19: Inez
(continued)

Case Presentation 19: Inez **Patient Impairment Profile**			
	Severity rating		
Impairment	**9/28/2001**	**10/19/2001**	**Endpoint goal**
1. Phobia	2	2	0
2. Dysphoric Mood	2	1	0
3. Social Withdrawal	2	1	0

Patient Objectives: Progress Update

To Be Addressed by Treatment Completion: 11/23/2001

(% = percent progress)

Phobia
Patient will verbalize
- Acceptance of the responsibility for coping with the Phobia **(75%)**
- Awareness of the potential links (via conditioned learning) between the Phobia and past (recent and/or remote) experience **(75%)**
- Coping response alternatives to phobic avoidance **(50%)**
- A plan of action to be taken should the Phobia exacerbate **(10%)**

Patient will demonstrate
- Participation in the prescribed treatment program **(100%)**
- Successful use of relaxation techniques in the presence of the feared stimuli (e.g., dogs shown on television, dogs in the park) **(25%)**
- Ability to pet dogs known to be friendly **(0%)**
- Elimination of the Phobia as evidenced by a normal-range score on the State-Trait Anxiety Inventory for Adults state scale while patient thinks about dogs **(initial score = 56; current score = 49; average score = 35.20)**
- A completed self-care (discharge) plan, including steps to be taken should the Phobia return **(0%)**

Dysphoric Mood
Patient will verbalize
- Acceptance of responsibility for coping with the Dysphoric Mood **(100%)**
- Statements about self that are realistically positive and hopeful rather than unrealistically negative **(75%)**
- Warning signs that the Dysphoric Mood is exacerbating **(75%)**
- A plan of action to be taken should the Dysphoric Mood exacerbate **(10%)**

(continued)

Patient will demonstrate
- Adherence to the prescribed treatment program **(100%)**
- Increased self-initiated and self-directed activities **(75%)**
- Elimination of Dysphoric Mood **(50%)**
- A completed self-care (discharge) plan, including steps to be taken should the Dysphoric Mood return or exacerbate **(0%)**

Social Withdrawal

Patient will verbalize
- Acceptance of the responsibility for coping with Social Withdrawal **(100%)**
- Awareness that Social Withdrawal can increase the severity of both Phobia and Dysphoric Mood **(100%)**
- Warning signs that the Social Withdrawal is exacerbating **(100%)**
- A plan of action to be taken should the Social Withdrawal exacerbate **(75%)**

Patient will demonstrate
- Participation in the prescribed treatment program **(100%)**
- Plans and activities to be initiated with her husband or friends at previous (i.e., before impairment onset) frequency levels **(100%)**
- Elimination of Social Withdrawal **(100%)**
- A completed self-care (discharge) plan, including steps to be taken should the Social Withdrawal return or exacerbate **(75%)**

Tracking Patient Progress **167**

Tracking Progress and Outcomes:
Study Questions—Inez

Instructions: *Read each of the questions below and circle the* most *correct response.*

1. According to the PIP system, if patient progress occurs over time, it must be noted *at least* by the following:

   a) a decrease in the severity rating of an impairment.
   b) an increase in the percent of progress toward meeting an objective.
   c) a and b.
   d) none of the above.

2. Inez's treatment plan states that the severity of her Phobia has remained destabilizing (severity of 2). This must imply that

   a) her Phobia still markedly compromises (30%–60%) her self-care functioning.
   b) she has made no progress toward resolving her Phobia.
   c) her Phobia has not worsened significantly.
   d) a and b.

3. Inez's Social Withdrawal is currently rated at a severity of 1. This can imply that

   a) she has made no progress regarding her Social Withdrawal.
   b) her Social Withdrawal still compromises (<30%) her self-care functioning.
   c) her Social Withdrawal is no longer present.
   d) b or c.

4. Inez has made no progress toward the objective of petting a friendly dog. If she never makes any progress toward this objective, this implies that

   a) it will be impossible for her Phobia to be repaired.
   b) this objective will not be suitable for retention as a measure of her progress toward repairing her Phobia.
   c) this objective should never have been included in her treatment plan.
   d) Inez's endpoint goal regarding her Phobia will need to be changed to a maintenance goal.

5. Inez's State-Trait Anxiety Inventory for Adults state scale score *while she thinks about dogs* has dropped from 56 to 49. If her score drops further to 40 (i.e., within the normal range), this will imply that

   a) her Phobia has been repaired and must receive a severity rating of 0.
   b) her treatment should no longer address her Phobia.
   c) she is currently meeting one of her objectives regarding her Phobia.
   d) a and b.

Turn the page for the answers to these questions.

Tracking Progress and Outcomes: Answers to Study Questions

1. Answer "b" is correct. A reduction in the severity rating of an impairment need not occur for progress to be noted (Answer "a"). Smaller yet significant changes can and should be reflected in the percentage of progress made toward accomplishing the objectives, even before any change in severity rating can be documented (Answer "c"). Changes in severity ratings, however, will be associated with improvement in meeting objectives, and the former cannot occur without the latter.

2. Answer "a" is correct. Severity ratings reflect the overall level of dysfunction regarding impairments. These ratings are sufficiently global, however (e.g., "30%–60%"), that improvement regarding specific objectives can occur without a resultant reduction in impairment severity (Answer "b"). Conversely, the dysfunction associated with an impairment can increase (e.g., from 30% to 40%) without a coinciding increase in its severity (Answer "c").

3. Answer "d" is correct. The fact that Inez's severity rating for Social Withdrawal has moved from a 2 to a 1 implies that she must have made progress (Answer "a"). A severity of 1 can, and typically does, imply that an impairment is still compromising self-care functioning (Answer "b"), but this is not always true. A severity of 1 can also denote that an impairment is no longer present in the specific case where that impairment is expected to return without continued treatment (Answer "c"). More commonly, however, impairment absence will be associated with a severity of 0, indicating not only the absence but also the repair of an impairment.

4. Answer "b" is correct. Objectives are selected as *expected* signs of progress toward the goal of impairment resolution. An impairment can sometimes be repaired without having all objectives met, however, just as the same destination can be reached by alternative routes (Answers "a" and "d"). Indeed, Inez was eventually able to return to her former level of functioning around dogs without ever petting one. She stated, "I could certainly pet a dog now if I needed to, but I'm still not a 'dog person,' and I have no desire to change my preference." The practitioner's original selection of this objective was still useful, however (Answer "c"). Initially informing Inez about "treatments that have helped those who fear snakes to hold them and those who fear dogs to pet them," instilled hope, increased motivation, and facilitated her progress.

5. Answer "c" is correct. The data supplied by standardized measures are useful, but they seldom if ever correspond exactly to the information about a given impairment (Answer "a"). In most cases, scale scores will reflect either more general (i.e., depression) or more specific (e.g., negative thinking) information than is expressed by a given impairment definition. Furthermore, even when both scale scores and severity ratings reflect normal functioning (Answer "b"), treatment can continue (see Answer 3 above).

The Discharge Summary

Documenting Treatment Course

In this chapter, we show how Patient Impairment Profile (PIP)–based treatment plans can provide the basis for documenting and summarizing treatment results. The two example cases are used to illustrate this last step in patient management. Then a final new case provides the clinician with an integrated view of the entire PIP system—from initial PIP to discharge summary.

Definitions

outcome The result of the performance or nonperformace of a process or processes of care.

patient outcome The individual-specific results of the performance or nonperformance of a process or processes of care; the unique effect of care on the patient's functionality and well-being.

Treatment may be terminated for various reasons (e.g., all treatment goals have been accomplished, the patient or clinician moves to a new location, the patient decides to discontinue). Whatever the cause of termination, an increasing number of behavioral managed care organizations are requesting a documented treatment summary. Current trends indicate that requests for such summaries will most likely become commonplace—if not the norm—in the near future.

Discharge summaries typically include the patient's identifying information, diagnosis (e.g., at treatment onset and cessation), some type of progress summary (e.g., length of treatment, remaining impairments and severity ratings, and status of objectives), and continuing care recommendations (e.g., a discharge plan, the practitioner's recommendations, the patient's stated plans). In addition, the reason for cessation of treatment is usually noted.

The PIP system facilitates the summarizing of treatment *outcome* because the majority of documentation required for such a summary is already contained in the patient's treatment plan. Specifically, the information provided by the initial PIP, goals, objectives, and interventions—and the updates of these data—combines with final descriptions of *patient outcome* to provide a comprehensive synopsis of treatment.

Documenting April's Treatment Course
(Case 11 Conclusion)

In accordance with the recommendations of the treatment team, April moved to an unlocked unit during the late afternoon of her third day of hospitalization. She continued to improve steadily, maintaining all terms of her contract. For example, she consistently arrived 5 minutes early for her medication and attended her group therapy sessions without negative incident. She also participated in occupational therapy and showed increasing insight regarding her recent Delusions and Psychotic Thought/Behavior. Furthermore, she was able to state a plan of action to take should she notice any worsening of these impairments: "I will tell my coordinator if any strange ideas or urges bother me." She also showed improvement in her Inadequate Self-Maintenance Skills, stating, "I feel even better, and I am able to be polite to others as I would like them to be to me."

The treatment team determined that April had met all her target objectives by the end of her sixth day. As a result of this progress, they agreed that she should be discharged from inpatient treatment the next morning and transferred back to the group home. The following discharge summary was documented:

The Discharge Summary: Documenting Treatment Course   171

Case Presentation 11: April
Discharge Summary: 4/16/2001

Diagnosis at intake

DSM-IV Axis I diagnosis: 295.10 Schizophrenia, disorganized type

DSM-IV Axis II diagnosis: None

Diagnosis at discharge

DSM-IV Axis I diagnosis: 295.10 Schizophrenia, disorganized type

DSM-IV Axis II diagnosis: None

Length of treatment

Inpatient treatment for 6 days (4/10/2001 to 4/16/2001)

Reason for treatment cessation

Target objectives met

Discharge plan

Transfer back to the group home for continued treatment.

Patient Impairment Profile				
	Severity rating			
Impairment	**4/10/2001**	**4/12/2001**	**4/16/2001**	**Interim goal**
1. Delusions (Nonparanoid)	4	2	1	2
2. Psychotic Thought/Behavior	3	3	1	2
3. Inadequate Self-Maintenance Skills	2	1	1	1
4. Educational Performance Deficit	2	2	2	2

Patient Objectives: Progress Summary

To Be Addressed by Discharge From Inpatient Setting to Group Home Setting: 4/16/2001

(*Target Objective—to be met 100%) (% = percent progress)

Delusions (Nonparanoid)

Patient will verbalize

- Awareness of the presence of Delusional thinking **(100%)**
- Acceptance of the responsibility for coping with the Delusions **(100%)**
- Precipitants for the Delusional thinking **(50%)**
- Warning signs that the Delusions are exacerbating **(50%)**
- * A plan of action to be taken should the Delusions exacerbate **(100%)**

Patient will demonstrate

- * Absence of Delusions for 72 hours **(100%)**
- Adherence to a prescribed treatment program **(100%)**
- * A completed self-care (discharge) plan, including steps to be taken should the Delusions return or exacerbate **(100%)**

Psychotic Thought/Behavior

Patient will verbalize

- Awareness of the presence of Psychotic Thought/Behavior **(100%)**
- Acceptance of the responsibility for coping with the Psychotic Thought/Behavior **(100%)**
- Precipitants for the Psychotic Thought/Behavior **(75%)**
- Warning signs that the Psychotic Thought/Behavior is exacerbating **(50%)**
- * A plan of action to be taken should the Psychotic Thought/Behavior exacerbate **(100%)**

Patient will demonstrate

- * Absence of Psychotic Thought/Behavior for 72 hours **(100%)**
- Adherence to prescribed treatment program **(100%)**
- * A completed self-care (discharge) plan, including steps to be taken should the Psychotic Thought/Behavior return or exacerbate **(100%)**

To Be Met by Completion of Treatment and Resumption of Semi-Independent Living: 6/18/2001

Delusions (Nonparanoid)

Patient will verbalize

Awareness that Delusions can resume without maintained adherence to a discharge plan **(75%)**

(continued)

Patient will demonstrate
- Maintained adherence to a self-care plan with maintained absence of Delusions **(25%)**

Psychotic Thought/Behavior

Patient will verbalize
- Awareness that Psychotic Thought/Behavior can resume without maintained adherence to a discharge plan **(75%)**

Patient will demonstrate
- Maintained adherence to a self-care plan with adequate management of Psychotic Thought/Behavior **(10%)**

Inadequate Self-Maintenance Skills

Patient will verbalize
- Awareness of the presence of Inadequate Self-Maintenance Skills **(100%)**
- Acceptance of the responsibility for coping with the Inadequate Self-Maintenance Skills **(100%)**
- Awareness of the dangers or adverse consequences of Inadequate Self-Maintenance Skills **(75%)**
- A plan of action to be taken should the Inadequate Self-Maintenance Skills exacerbate **(50%)**

Patient will demonstrate
- Adherence to a prescribed treatment program **(100%)**
- Adequate management of the Inadequate Self-Maintenance Skills **(75%)**
- A completed self-care (discharge) plan, including steps to be taken should the Inadequate Self-Maintenance Skills return or exacerbate **(50%)**

Educational Performance Deficit

Patient will verbalize
- Awareness of the Educational Performance Deficit and its negative effect **(0%)**
- Acceptance of the responsibility for coping with the Educational Performance Deficit **(0%)**
- Willingness to participate in an Educational Performance Deficit assessment and remediation program **(0%)**

Patient will demonstrate
- Participation in a remediation program **(0%)**

April's current discharge summary indicates that she met all of her interim goals and even exceeded her goal regarding both Delusions and Psychotic Thought/Behavior (severity of 1 versus 2). This summary also shows the progress she made in her objectives. The fact that none of her impairments were completely repaired, however, supports the discharge plan of ongoing care. She is being transferred back to the group home, but her original treatment plan also proposed that continued treatment would involve facilitating her transition from the group home back to her semi-independent apartment. Thus, April's goals and objectives—with her entire treatment plan—now will need to be reassessed by the primary provider to whom her case is being transferred.

Because this new practitioner also uses the PIP system, treatment plan development will simply involve beginning where April's discharge summary ended. Specifically, most relevant information (e.g., current diagnosis, PIP) can be easily acquired from April's inpatient discharge summary. Of course, treatment goals must be reassessed because those identified during her inpatient hospitalization were only interim goals. Now, maintenance or endpoint goals must be identified, and objectives need to be modified, added, or deleted accordingly. At the cessation of treatment, another discharge summary will be generated.

The above discussion of April's ongoing treatment illustrates many of the advantages of the PIP system as a universal impairment nomenclature, which can be used by all mental health professionals. When this system is used at every level of treatment within a managed care network, its full benefits can be realized. Such benefits include continuity of documentation, reduced redundancy of administrative work, succinct transfer of relevant information between treatment settings, and generation of comprehensive data for use in quality measurement and improvement.

Documenting Billy's Treatment Course
(Case 12 Conclusion)

Billy's parents called to cancel his fourth session because Billy "caught a cold." They reported, however, that Billy was "doing much better emotionally. He's virtually back to his cheerful self." They agreed to continue working with his star chart and regular voiding schedule. During the next four sessions, Billy showed continued progress regarding his Enuresis. Furthermore, use of role-playing for forgiveness allowed him to verbalize and enact "what to do if I feel the 'guilty uh-oh' feelings." During the fifth week, he successfully spent the night at his grandmother's house without incident. During the sixth week, Billy did have two bed-wetting episodes 3 days apart, but he was able to minimize these by successful use of the alarm.

The clinician assessed Billy's Pathological Guilt, based on his progress, as repaired (having met all objectives). The clinician also considered Billy's Enuresis to be repaired (severity of 0) because Billy was now successfully self-managing this impairment, and his bed-wetting had declined to a nonpathological frequency. Thus, a discharge plan was prescribed, treatment was completed with the seventh session (eighth week), and the following discharge summary was documented:

The Discharge Summary: Documenting Treatment Course 175

Case Presentation 12: Billy
Discharge Summary: 8/20/2001

Diagnosis at intake

DSM-IV Axis I diagnosis: 307.6 Enuresis, nocturnal only

DSM-IV Axis II diagnosis: None

Diagnosis at discharge

DSM-IV Axis I diagnosis: None

DSM-IV Axis II diagnosis: None

Length of treatment

Seven weekly outpatient therapy sessions (7/2/2001 to 8/20/2001), with one cancellation during the fourth week

Reason for treatment cessation

Impairments repaired

Discharge plan

The patient will use the enuresis alarm for 6 additional weeks, followed by 2 weeks of gradual use reduction (e.g., every other night), and discontinuation thereafter.
Recurrence of Enuresis thereafter will be addressed by resuming alarm use for only 2 nights after any such episode.

Patient Impairment Profile			
	Severity rating		
Impairment	**7/2/2001**	**7/16/2001**	**8/20/2001**	**Endpoint goal**
1. Enuresis	1	1	0	0
2. Pathological Guilt	1	1	0	0

176   Casebook for Managing Managed Care

Patient Objectives: Progress Summary
To Be Addressed by Treatment Completion: 8/20/2001

(% = percent progress)

Enuresis

Patient will verbalize

- Awareness of the presence of Enuresis **(100%)**
- Acceptance of the responsibility for coping with the Enuresis **(100%)**
- Willingness to participate in the treatment of Enuresis **(100%)**
- A plan of action to be taken should the Enuresis exacerbate **(100%)**

Patient will demonstrate

- Adherence to a prescribed treatment program **(100%)**
- Elimination of Enuresis **(100%)**
- A completed self-care (discharge) plan, including steps to be taken should the Enuresis exacerbate **(100%)**

Pathological Guilt

Patient will verbalize

- Awareness of the Pathological Guilt and its current adverse consequences (e.g., generalized anxiety) **(100%)**
- Willingness to participate in the treatment of Pathological Guilt **(100%)**

Patient will demonstrate

- Elimination of Pathological Guilt as evidenced by cessation of repetitive apologizing behavior **(100%)**
- A completed self-care (discharge) plan, including steps to be taken should the Pathological Guilt exacerbate **(100%)**

Step 7: Documenting Treatment Course

One new case follows. As in Chapter 7, you will create an Impairment Inventory (Steps 1 and 2) and then create a PIP (Step 3). Goals, objectives (Step 4), and interventions (Step 5) are presented next. Then, patient progress (Step 6) is reported, followed by a discharge summary (Step 7) outlining the patient's status at treatment cessation. Based on this collective information, multiple-choice questions are then presented to facilitate integration of treatment course documentation (i.e., impairments, severities, the PIP, goals, objectives, interventions, and progress). This final new case provides the clinician with the opportunity to integrate all components of the PIP system when documenting the entire course of treatment. Once again, please read the vignette and imagine that you are actually interviewing the identified patient.

The Discharge Summary: Documenting Treatment Course

Notes

Turn the page for the next case.

178   **Casebook for Managing Managed Care**

Case Presentation 20

"Vince"

Reason for Referral

Vince, a 73-year-old African American man, was referred to you for evaluation by his physician. He is complaining of having difficulty sleeping. In addition, his physician feels that he is having trouble adapting to his new treatment regimen. This concern is supported by his gradual but significant weight gain (15 lbs) over the past 8 weeks after he received the diagnosis of "late-onset diabetes." Vince's sleeping difficulties also began after receiving this diagnosis. He complains of almost always having trouble falling asleep initially and also after waking up to use the bathroom. He feels that the sleep loss may explain why "I always feel drained." His physician states that Vince's diabetes is mild and can be controlled with oral medication. Still, the physician is concerned that Vince's "forgetting" (once or twice per week) to take his daily pills could present a medical risk in the future, especially if his condition worsens. You interview Vince and obtain the following information:

History

Vince reports that he has "never been sick a day in my life" until the onset of his diabetes. He is "happily married" and enjoys spending time with his grandchildren. He states that receiving this diagnosis "made me face the fact that I am not getting any younger." For the last month, he has found himself continually "feeling blue" and preoccupied with morbid issues, especially at bedtime (e.g., death, estate planning, his own parents' deaths 15 and 17 years earlier). This has made it hard for him to fall asleep. "Then I started waking up a lot, too, to use the bathroom; but the doctor says I just have to get used to that as part of this awful disease." He describes his wife as "very supportive" but adds, "I don't like to bother her with this. She's got enough problems with her bad back." He further states, "I have always taken care of her, and it feels strange to have the shoe on the other foot."

Clinical Presentation

Vince presents as a well-dressed, well-groomed, obese man of average height. He appears calm and attempts to be cheerful but does become tearful at times. He is alert and articulate, maintains good eye contact, and is generally pleasant—even when recounting his current difficulties. When questioned, Vince admits that "I do forget those silly pills quite often." He also admits that his forgetfulness "is probably due to my not wanting to accept this." He further explains that "life would be terrific if I just didn't have this disease to deal with. I know I should watch my weight, but a few sweets now and then help me feel better. I guess I should be thankful for having had such good health up until now, but I just can't seem to help being upset about all this."

Assessment Assumptions

Sleeping difficulties and weight gain are related to, but not caused by, the medical condition. No substance abuse or eating disorder is present. All factors not explicitly mentioned above have been ruled out. In your waiting room, Vince completed the Center for Epidemiologic Studies—Depressed Mood Scale (Radloff 1977). His score was 2 standard deviations above the mean, reflecting significant symptomatology.

> **DSM-IV Axis I diagnosis**: 296.21 Major depression, single episode, mild
> **DSM-IV Axis II diagnosis:** None

Identify the impairments and rate their severities on the next page.

The Discharge Summary: Documenting Treatment Course   **179**

Steps 1 & 2:
Identifying Impairments and Rating Severity

Instructions: *List **all the impairments**, with their respective **severity ratings**. After each, cite **behavioral evidence (statements/actions)** that supports your choices of both impairments and severities. List the impairments that refer **only to Vince**. Remember that information **not** mentioned should be assumed to be **nonapplicable** to this patient (e.g., no organic pathology is present). Assume that all symptoms and/or relevant information are reported in the case description.*

Impairment Inventory	
Impairment	**Severity rating**
1.	
Behavioral evidence:	
2.	
Behavioral evidence:	
3.	
Behavioral evidence:	
4.	
Behavioral evidence:	
5.	
Behavioral evidence:	

Turn the page for Impairment Inventory and severity rating answers.

Impairment Inventory	
(Impairments are listed chronologically as they appear in the vignette.)	
Impairment	**Severity rating**
1. Altered Sleep *(noncritical)*	**2** *(Destabilizing)*
Behavioral evidence: Vince almost always has difficulty falling asleep. "Then I started waking up a lot, too…but the doctor says I just have to get used to that as part of this awful disease." "I always feel drained."	
2. Medical Treatment Noncompliance *(noncritical)*	**2** *(Destabilizing)*
Behavioral evidence: He has gained 15 pounds. "I know I should watch my weight, but a few sweets now and then help me feel better." He is "forgetting" (once or twice per week) to take his daily pills.	
3. Concomitant Medical Condition *(critical)*	**2** *(Destabilizing)*
Behavioral evidence: He received a diagnosis of "late-onset diabetes" 8 weeks ago. His physician states that Vince's diabetes is mild and can be controlled with oral medication.	
4. Dysphoric Mood *(critical)*	**2** *(Destabilizing)*
Behavioral evidence: For the last month, he has been continually "feeling blue" and preoccupied with morbid issues, especially at bedtime (e.g., death, estate planning, his own parents' deaths). He attempts to be cheerful but becomes tearful at times. "I just can't seem to help being upset about all this." His score on the Center for Epidemiologic Studies—Depressed Mood Scale was 2 standard deviations above the mean, reflecting significant symptomatology.	

Common Errors

Eating Disorder: Vince's recent weight gain is related to—but not caused by—his Concomitant Medical Condition. His eating habits have become problematic because they violate his increased dietary restrictions. As such, these habits are also part of his medical treatment noncompliance, and his eating behavior can be addressed with respect to this latter impairment in his PIP. Thus, although he is (and has been) obese, Vince does not have a "gross disturbance in eating behavior."

Medical Risk Factor: Some of Vince's behaviors involve medical risks (e.g., his failure to take his medicine), but he does not require any mental health interventions (e.g., electroconvulsive therapy) that might themselves cause an "adverse reaction or other medical complication." Note that Medical Risk Factor is distinguished from Concomitant Medical Condition.

Create the Patient Impairment Profile (PIP) on the next page.

The Discharge Summary: Documenting Treatment Course   **181**

Step 3: Creating the Patient Impairment Profile

Instructions: *Now, select those impairments from Vince's Impairment Inventory that will be the current focus of treatment. List them with their respective severity ratings on the Patient Impairment Profile below. List the impairments in **prioritized order.** Then, in the space below, write your rationale for your ranking of each. Remember that information **not** mentioned should be assumed to be **nonapplicable** to this patient.*

Patient Impairment Profile	
Impairment	**Severity rating**
1.	
2.	
3.	
4.	

1. Prioritization rationale:
2. Prioritization rationale:
3. Prioritization rationale:
4. Prioritization rationale:

Turn the page for prioritized PIP answers.

Case Presentation 20: Vince	
Patient Impairment Profile	
Impairment	**Severity rating**
1. Dysphoric Mood	2
2. Concomitant Medical Condition	2
3. Medical Treatment Noncompliance	2

1. Prioritization rationale: This impairment appears to be the cause of Vince's Medical Treatment Noncompliance that could "present a medical risk in the future." His Dysphoric Mood also may be exacerbating his Altered Sleep (via thinking about morbid issues at bedtime), as well as his obesity (because sweets help him "feel better").

2. Prioritization rationale: Vince's diabetes must be effectively managed (e.g., with the help of a physician), even if he fails to comply with mental health treatment, to prevent worsening of this condition. (His Altered Sleep most likely will be addressed by successfully treating this impairment and his Dysphoric Mood.)

3. Prioritization rationale: Helping Vince to master self-management of his medical conditions will not only prevent additional medical risks but also ensure an optimal quality of life.

Common Error

Concomitant Medical Condition: Some practitioners might want to give this impairment top priority in the PIP because of the serious risks involved in failure to manage diabetes. Note, however, that a mental health practitioner will view such illnesses primarily as they relate to psychological versus physical functioning. (A physician is already treating Vince's diabetes and will continue to do so.) Thus, viewing Vince's Concomitant Medical Condition as it relates to mental health results in prioritizing it after his Dysphoric Mood in his PIP. Specifically, if not for his Dysphoric Mood—and his apparent resulting Medical Treatment Noncompliance (e.g., "forgetting" to take medication)—a physician would have remained solely responsible for this patient. Note that *impairments in the Impairment Inventory describe patient dysfunctions relating to mental health concerns.*

The Discharge Summary: Documenting Treatment Course   **183**

Step 4: Identifying Goals and Objectives

Because Vince described his wife as "very supportive" but also did not "want to bother her with this," the clinician believed that treatment would probably be most effective if she accompanied him to future sessions. By doing so, the practitioner hoped to provide Vince with a rationale for asking his wife for help, as part of "doctor's orders." Thus, weekly individual psychotherapy sessions were prescribed, and Vince's wife was invited as a "consultant." A concurrent referral to a local diabetes support group was made. Short-term outpatient treatment was viewed as sufficient, with the expectation that Vince (and his wife) would be able to continue in the support group after treatment completion. The initial goals based on Vince's PIP thus were also cited as endpoint goals. The following goals and objectives are *suggestions* only:

Treatment Plan for Case Presentation 20: Vince

Case Presentation 20: Vince Patient Impairment Profile		
	Severity rating	
Impairment	**3/9/2001**	**Endpoint goal**
1. Dysphoric Mood	2	0
2. Concomitant Medical Condition	2	0
3. Medical Treatment Noncompliance	2	0

Patient Objectives
To Be Addressed by Treatment Completion: 4/20/2001

Dysphoric Mood

Patient will verbalize
- Acceptance of the responsibility for coping with the Dysphoric Mood
- Statements about the self and diabetes that are realistically positive and hopeful rather than unrealistically negative
- Warning signs that the Dysphoric Mood is exacerbating
- A plan of action to be taken should the Dysphoric Mood exacerbate

Patient will demonstrate
- Adherence to the prescribed treatment program
- Reduced morbid thinking at or near bedtime
- Elimination of the Dysphoric Mood as evidenced by a normal-range score on the Center for Epidemiologic Studies—Depressed Mood Scale
- A completed self-care (discharge) plan, including steps to be taken should the Dysphoric Mood return or exacerbate

(continued)

Concomitant Medical Condition

Patient will verbalize

- Acceptance of the responsibility for the management of the Concomitant Medical Condition
- Thoughts and feelings regarding the Concomitant Medical Condition
- Warning signs that the Concomitant Medical Condition is exacerbating
- A plan of action to be taken should the Concomitant Medical Condition exacerbate

Patient will demonstrate

- Adherence to the treatment regimen for the Concomitant Medical Condition as prescribed by his physician (e.g., medication)
- Adequate management of the Concomitant Medical Condition
- A completed self-care (discharge) plan, including steps to be taken should the Concomitant Medical Condition return or exacerbate

Medical Treatment Noncompliance

Patient will verbalize

- Acceptance of the need for long-term medical treatment compliance
- Thoughts and feelings regarding the Medical Treatment Noncompliance
- Warning signs that the Medical Treatment Noncompliance is exacerbating
- A plan of action to be taken should medical treatment compliance falter or deteriorate

Patient will demonstrate

- Successful use of a medication schedule checklist to eliminate "forgetting" behavior
- Adherence to the prescribed medical treatment program
- A completed self-care (discharge) plan, including steps to be taken should medical treatment compliance falter or deteriorate

Step 5: Selecting Interventions

Based on the previously discussed assessment, diagnosis, and treatment modalities, the practitioner chose the interventions listed below. Given the various depressive symptoms associated with Vince's Dysphoric Mood (see Appendix A), treatment included antidepressant medication. This treatment was administered particularly because these symptoms were potentially exacerbating Vince's Medical Treatment Noncompliance. In addition, Vince reported a positive family history for major depression (his mother), signaling another prognostic indicator for antidepressant use. The clinician prescribed Prozac (fluoxetine) because of its lack of diabetes-complicating side effects (e.g., weight gain) that can occur with some other antidepressants (e.g., tricyclics). Vince's wife enthusiastically agreed to attend the therapy sessions. Remember, however, that—as the identified patient—only Vince provided the basis for the PIP, objectives, and goals. The following interventions, representing the continuation of Vince's treatment plan described above, are *suggestions* only:

The Discharge Summary: Documenting Treatment Course   185

Treatment Plan for Case Presentation 20: Vince
(continued)

Practitioner Interventions

Dysphoric Mood

Psychopharmacotherapy:
- Treat Dysphoric Mood with Prozac (fluoxetine) 20 mg/day in the morning.

Individual therapy:
- Validate Vince's thoughts and feelings regarding his Dysphoric Mood.
- Suggest that Vince identify all positive facets of his life that are not deleteriously affected by his diabetes.
- Suggest that Vince keep a nightly journal—before bedtime—listing as many positive aspects (e.g., events, insights) of that day as he can recall.

Concomitant Medical Condition

Psychopharmacotherapy:
- Assess the appropriateness of medication for Vince's sleep difficulty, as it relates to his Concomitant Medical Condition.

Individual therapy:
- Validate his thoughts and feelings regarding his Concomitant Medical Condition.
- Educate Vince about the mental health factors (e.g., stress, coping) influencing his Concomitant Medical Condition (e.g., eating to alleviate stress, "forgetting" his medicine).
- Clarify the nature of Vince's apparent resistance to having his wife help with his healthcare.
- Suggest that Vince consider drinking no fluids 90 minutes before bedtime to reduce his need to void at night.
- Initiate relaxation training and suggest that Vince use his relaxation tape on waking at night.
- Encourage Vince to join the local diabetes support group.

Medical Treatment Noncompliance

Individual therapy:
- Validate Vince's thoughts and feelings regarding his Medical Treatment Noncompliance.
- Suggest that Vince consider the long-term advantages (for himself and his wife) versus the short-term disadvantages of medical treatment compliance.
- Encourage Vince to make and use a medication schedule checklist to help eliminate "forgetting" behavior.

Note that an intervention listed under one impairment can be equally important for the resolution of other impairments. In Vince's case, although the practitioner listed diabetes support group attendance under Concomitant Medical Condition (see preceding page), it was viewed as relevant to each of his impairments. As stated previously, matching interventions with impairments is less crucial than choosing appropriate interventions overall for a given patient.

Step 6: Tracking Progress

During the intake, the clinician addressed Vince's concern that he "not bother" his wife with his distress. Vince responded favorably to the suggestion that it would help him and his wife if she joined him for therapy sessions. The clinician also encouraged Vince to verbalize his thoughts and feelings about his impairments. Vince focused on his recurring morbid thoughts of his own parents' deaths. He revealed, "I feel like both my parents died before I was ready to be the oldest generation, and now I could do the same to my kids." He also elaborated his feelings about having "never been sick a day in [his] life." He remarked, "Now that I am sick, it feels like I am a lot closer to death, and I haven't spent much time thinking about such things." Finally, he confessed, "I guess I feel a bit guilty because my wife has been on me about my weight for years, and maybe my weight is a cause of my diabetes." The clinician validated Vince's thoughts and feelings, suggesting that therapy could provide a "safe place" to explore these issues. The clinician also began to educate Vince about ways to manage his diabetes successfully. Vince remarked, "I wish my doctor had spent more time telling me the good news, like you have, instead of the bad news about all the things I will probably have to get used to." The clinician suggested that a local diabetes support group could provide Vince with additional helpful information "from people who have walked the same path." Vince agreed to attend one meeting to "check it out." Finally, the clinician also educated him regarding Prozac and the importance of taking his medications as prescribed.

In the second session, the clinician asked Vince's wife for her impressions of how Vince was doing. She reported that "Vince does really seem down in the dumps about this, and he doesn't seem to want any help from me, which upsets me." In response, Vince told his wife that he felt she already had "enough to cope with, what with your back and all." The clinician facilitated the ensuing conversation, in which Vince's wife clarified that she was glad to be able to help and support Vince "for once, after all these years." Vince seemed relieved and stated that this was "just one more proof that I married the right girl." The clinician suggested that Vince might find it helpful to verbalize his feelings about his diabetes to his wife whenever he felt stressed rather than keep them to himself. Vince's wife concurred, adding, "It's only fair, since he's had to listen to me complain about my back for years now." Based on Vince's report of continued sleep-onset difficulties—and given his age—Restoril (temazepam 15 mg at bedtime) was prescribed for the next 3 nights, followed by the same dose every other night thereafter. Altered Sleep was also added to the PIP. The clinician educated Vince about good sleep hygiene and gave him a relaxation tape and literature. Vince agreed to use the tape once during the day and once before bedtime.

Vince came alone to the third session because his wife had a conflicting appointment. He had attended the diabetes support group with her that week, however, and stated that "they are a really great group of people, and some of them even know what it is like to be over 70!" He added, "I don't know whether it's talking to you or taking that Prozac, but I think I am feeling a bit better!" The clinician asked Vince about his "forgetting" to take his medication, and Vince reported that he was still doing so "only once in a while and a lot less than before." He added, "Funny, but it's easier to remember three different pills than just one!" The clinician encouraged Vince to make a medication

The Discharge Summary: Documenting Treatment Course   **187**

schedule checklist to help eliminate this problem. Vince then raised the issue of his morbid thoughts, reporting that "I am falling asleep okay now, but I still find myself thinking about death at times." Vince was then encouraged to verbalize his fears of "leaving my kids behind like I was left." The clinician encouraged Vince to consider talking to his children about this concern soon, even though he might have many years left to live. Vince agreed that this might help him with this concern. The clinician also suggested that Vince begin a "blessings" journal to be written in just before bed, as a constructive way to avoid ruminating on morbid thoughts. Finally, Vince was instructed to discontinue the Restoril, but to continue using his relaxation tape before bedtime.

During the fourth session, Vince reported, "I really feel like I am making progress, like I have new hope about all this." His wife added that she noticed "a positive change in his spirits; he's not down as much anymore, and he has even encouraged some of the others at the support group." When asked about taking his medications, however, Vince responded sheepishly that he had not yet made the schedule checklist. He also admitted forgetting his diabetes medication two times during the week. When questioned further, Vince replied, "Well, I have been feeling a bit better so I guess I have been wondering if—just maybe—I don't have this stupid disease after all. Besides, what if I had it but I've gotten over it?" The clinician responded by encouraging Vince to verbalize his maintained feelings of frustration about "being stuck with this for the rest of my life." The clinician then encouraged Vince to consider focusing more on aspects of his physical health that he could change, such as his weight. Vince agreed to make his medication schedule checklist when he went home, and he would try to be more careful about his diet. He also reported that he was continuing to fall asleep more quickly both at bedtime and after waking to use the bathroom.

Based on this information, Vince's PIP-based treatment plan was updated as follows:

Treatment Plan for Case Presentation 20: Vince
(continued)

Case Presentation 20: Vince Patient Impairment Profile			
	Severity rating		
Impairment	3/9/2001	3/30/2001	Endpoint goal
1. Dysphoric Mood	2	1	0
2. Concomitant Medical Condition	2	1	0
3. Medical Treatment Noncompliance	2	1	0
4. Altered Sleep (added 3/16/2001)	—	1	0

Patient Objectives: Progress Update

To Be Addressed by Treatment Completion: 4/20/2001

(% = percent progress)

Dysphoric Mood

Patient will verbalize

- Acceptance of the responsibility for coping with the Dysphoric Mood **(100%)**
- Statements about the self and diabetes that are realistically positive and hopeful rather than unrealistically negative **(50%)**
- Warning signs that the Dysphoric Mood is exacerbating **(25%)**
- A plan of action to be taken should the Dysphoric Mood exacerbate **(0%)**

Patient will demonstrate

- Adherence to the prescribed treatment program **(100%)**
- Reduced morbid thinking at or near bedtime **(50%)**
- Elimination of Dysphoric Mood as evidenced by a normal-range score on the Center for Epidemiologic Studies—Depressed Mood Scale **(initial score = 20; current score = 12; normal range [Caucasian] = 7.94 to 9.25)**
- A completed self-care (discharge) plan, including steps to be taken should the Dysphoric Mood return or exacerbate **(0%)**

Concomitant Medical Condition

Patient will verbalize

- Acceptance of the responsibility for the management of the Concomitant Medical Condition **(80%)**
- Thoughts and feelings regarding the Concomitant Medical Condition **(100%)**
- Warning signs that the Concomitant Medical Condition is exacerbating **(100%)**
- A plan of action to be taken should the Concomitant Medical Condition exacerbate **(100%)**

Patient will demonstrate

- Adherence to the treatment regimen for the Concomitant Medical Condition as prescribed by his physician (e.g., medication) **(80%)**
- Adequate management of the Concomitant Medical Condition **(80%)**
- A completed self-care (discharge) plan, including steps to be taken should the Concomitant Medical Condition return or exacerbate **(50%)**

Medical Treatment Noncompliance

Patient will verbalize

- Acceptance of the need for long-term medical treatment compliance **(75%)**
- Thoughts and feelings regarding the Medical Treatment Noncompliance **(100%)**
- Warning signs that the Medical Treatment Noncompliance is exacerbating **(75%)**
- A plan of action to be taken should medical treatment compliance falter or deteriorate **(100%)**

(continued)

Patient will demonstrate
- Successful use of a medication schedule checklist to eliminate "forgetting" behavior **(0%)**
- Adherence to the prescribed medical treatment program **(75%)**
- A completed self-care (discharge) plan, including steps to be taken should medical treatment compliance falter or deteriorate **(50%)**

Altered Sleep
Patient will verbalize:
- Acceptance of responsibility for coping with the Altered Sleep **(100%)**
- Awareness that Altered Sleep can increase the severity of both Concomitant Medical Condition and Dysphoric Mood **(100%)**
- Warning signs that the Altered Sleep is exacerbating **(100%)**
- A plan of action to be taken should the Altered Sleep return or worsen **(100%)**

Patient will demonstrate:
- Participation in the prescribed treatment program **(100%)**
- Elimination of Altered Sleep **(100%)**
- A completed self-care (discharge) plan, including steps to be taken should the Altered Sleep return or exacerbate **(75%)**

Vince's treatment progress update provides evidence supporting not only his need for continued treatment but also his significant improvement. As has been stated previously, remember that both of these facets of the progress update are equally important in communicating the clinical rationale for continued treatment.

Step 7: Documenting Vince's Treatment Course
(Case 20 Conclusion)

Over the next 3 weeks, Vince continued to make progress in reducing his impairments. He was attending the diabetes support group regularly and described it as "very rewarding, not only for the support I get but for how I feel when I can encourage somebody else." During the fifth session, he reported having talked with his kids about his death concerns (i.e., his fear of leaving them "unprepared"). Two days earlier, the extended family had gone to Easter church services together, and this conversation occurred afterward at the family barbecue. Vince stated, "The topic just came up naturally, and I was able to really talk to my kids. I haven't done that since they were little." He added that he was considering "going back to church, which makes it easier to talk to the Man Upstairs." When questioned further, he reported that he was no longer having morbid thoughts "now that death isn't the 'taboo topic.' Besides, I'm planning on sticking around for a good while!"

Vince also reported that he had completed and was successfully using his medication schedule checklist. His sleep-onset difficulties were "gone," and he had "a lot less trouble getting back to sleep when I wake up in the middle of the night. Not drinking before bed does seem to help too." Furthermore, his wife reported that "Vince seems to be accepting his diabetes now and taking it in stride." Vince agreed, stating, "I've been through tougher things than this."

The sixth session focused on helping Vince to develop his own self-care plans, emphasizing his need to recognize the warning signs of impairment resurgence. Vince remarked that he planned to share his "warning signs" with the diabetes support group members "because we could all use help with the stress." Regarding his need to avoid sweets, Vince confessed, "I still have a little trouble with this one, but I think I'm getting there." Vince agreed to continue monitoring his diet with the assistance of his physician. His physician would monitor Vince's Prozac dosage and/or supervise discontinuation. Based on his overall progress, it was agreed that the seventh session would represent Vince's "promotion to self-care."

In the seventh session, termination issues were addressed, and Vince read a letter he had written of his own accord during the week. It was a note of thanks to the clinician "for helping me out big time to get through a hard time." Vince also reported that he had volunteered to be the diabetes support group host during the upcoming month and that he and his wife had met some new friends at church. The clinician congratulated Vince on his "promotion to self-care," and the case was closed.

Based on all previous information about Vince, the following discharge summary was documented:

Case Presentation 20: Vince

Discharge Summary: 4/20/2001

Diagnosis at intake

DSM-IV Axis I diagnosis: 296.21 Major depression, single episode, mild

DSM-IV Axis II diagnosis: None

Diagnosis at discharge

DSM-IV Axis I diagnosis: None

DSM-IV Axis II diagnosis: None

Length of treatment

Seven weekly outpatient therapy sessions (3/9/2001 to 4/20/2001)

Reason for treatment cessation

Impairments repaired

Discharge plan

Vince will continue to receive treatment for diabetes from his physician, who will also monitor his diet and use of Prozac. Vince will continue to attend the diabetes support group, and he will use his relaxation tape as needed.

The Discharge Summary: Documenting Treatment Course **191**

Patient Impairment Profile				
	Severity rating			
Impairment	**3/9/2001**	**3/30/2001**	**4/20/2001**	**Endpoint goal**
1. Dysphoric Mood	2	1	0	0
2. Concomitant Medical Condition	2	1	0	0
3. Medical Treatment Noncompliance	2	1	0	0
4. Altered Sleep (added 3/16/2001)	—	1	0	0

Patient Objectives: Progress Summary

To Be Addressed by Treatment Completion: 4/20/2001

(% = percent progress)

Dysphoric Mood

Patient will verbalize
- Acceptance of the responsibility for coping with the Dysphoric Mood **(100%)**
- Statements about the self and diabetes that are realistically positive and hopeful rather than unrealistically negative **(100%)**
- Warning signs that the Dysphoric Mood is exacerbating **(100%)**
- A plan of action to be taken should the Dysphoric Mood exacerbate **(100%)**

Patient will demonstrate
- Adherence to the prescribed treatment program **(100%)**
- Reduction in morbid thinking at or near bedtime **(100%)**
- Elimination of Dysphoric Mood as evidenced by a normal-range score on the Center for Epidemiologic Studies—Depressed Mood Scale **(initial score = 20; current score = 7; normal range [Caucasian] = 7.94 to 9.25)**
- A completed self-care (discharge) plan, including steps to be taken should the Dysphoric Mood return or exacerbate **(100%)**

(continued)

Concomitant Medical Condition

Patient will verbalize

- Acceptance of the responsibility for the management of the Concomitant Medical Condition **(100%)**
- Thoughts and feelings regarding the Concomitant Medical Condition **(100%)**
- Warning signs that the Concomitant Medical Condition is exacerbating **(100%)**
- A plan of action to be taken should the Concomitant Medical Condition exacerbate **(100%)**

Patient will demonstrate

- Adherence to the treatment regimen for the Concomitant Medical Condition as prescribed by his physician (e.g., medication) **(90%; still violating dietary restrictions)**
- Adequate management of the Concomitant Medical Condition **(95%; dietary violations are only a minor problem)**
- A completed self-care (discharge) plan, including steps to be taken should the Concomitant Medical Condition return or exacerbate **(100%)**

Medical Treatment Noncompliance

Patient will verbalize

- Acceptance of the need for long-term medical treatment compliance **(100%)**
- Thoughts and feelings regarding the Medical Treatment Noncompliance **(100%)**
- Warning signs that the Medical Treatment Noncompliance is exacerbating **(100%)**
- A plan of action to be taken should medical treatment compliance falter or deteriorate **(100%)**

Patient will demonstrate

- Successful use of a medication schedule checklist to eliminate "forgetting" behavior **(100%)**
- Adherence to the prescribed medical treatment program **(100%)**
- A completed self-care (discharge) plan, including steps to be taken should medical treatment compliance falter or deteriorate **(100%)**

Altered Sleep

Patient will verbalize:

- Acceptance of responsibility for coping with the Altered Sleep **(100%)**
- Awareness that Altered Sleep can increase the severity of both Concomitant Medical Condition and Dysphoric Mood **(100%)**
- Warning signs that the Altered Sleep is exacerbating **(100%)**
- A plan of action to be taken should the Altered Sleep return or worsen **(100%)**

Patient will demonstrate:

- Participation in the prescribed treatment program **(100%)**
- Elimination of Altered Sleep **(100%)**
- A completed self-care (discharge) plan, including steps to be taken should the Altered Sleep return or exacerbate **(100%)**

The Discharge Summary: Documenting Treatment Course   **193**

Documenting Treatment Course:
Study Questions—Vince

Instructions: *Read each of the questions below and circle the* most *correct response.*

1. According to the PIP system, complete repair of impairments must include the following:

   a) notation of 100% progress for all objectives on a discharge summary.
   b) severity ratings of 1 or lower on all impairments in the PIP.
   c) severity ratings of 0 on all impairments in the PIP.
   d) a and c.

2. Vince's discharge summary documents no DSM-IV diagnoses at treatment completion. When no diagnosis is reported, this implies that

   a) all impairment severity ratings must be 0.
   b) all objectives must reflect 100% progress ratings.
   c) a and b.
   d) none of the above.

3. Vince's Concomitant Medical Condition received a final severity rating of 0 on his discharge summary PIP. This must imply that

   a) he has made 100% progress on every objective regarding this impairment.
   b) he no longer has diabetes.
   c) he is self-managing his illness, and it causes him no undue psychological distress.
   d) absolutely no behavioral concerns regarding his Concomitant Medical Condition remain.

4. In the PIP presented in a discharge summary, the following should *always* be documented:

   a) goals.
   b) endpoint goals.
   c) interim goals.
   d) a, b, and c.

5. If Vince had still been "forgetting" his medication frequently at the time treatment was discontinued, this would have been noted in his discharge summary by

   a) a severity rating of 1 or higher for Medical Treatment Noncompliance.
   b) a DSM-IV diagnosis indicating current pathology.
   c) a and b.
   d) none of the above.

Turn the page for the answers to these questions.

Documenting Treatment Course:
Answers to Study Questions

1. Answer "c" is correct. Not all objectives regarding a given impairment need to note 100% progress (Answer "a"), provided that the impairment is repaired or nonpathological. Ideally, all objectives should note 100% progress, but this does not always occur. In Vince's case, two objectives regarding Concomitant Medical Condition (concerning proper dietary behavior) were not completely accomplished. These minor issues, however, were not preventing adequate diabetes self-management, nor were they causing him distress. In contrast, a severity rating of 1 never denotes complete impairment repair (Answer "b").

2. Answer "d" is correct. One or more impairments can still be present in the absence of a DSM-IV diagnosis, because their presence is not necessarily sufficient to meet the criteria for any DSM-IV diagnosis (Answer "a"). Of course, then, all objectives need not be accomplished either (Answer "b"). We hope that managed care organizations in the future will recognize that the need for treatment can sometimes occur in the absence of a DSM-IV diagnosis, just as they currently recognize that not all diagnoses warrant treatment (e.g., see "Case Presentation 10" in Chapter 4).

3. Answer "c" is correct. As stated above (see Answer 1), not all objectives will necessarily reflect 100% progress regarding a given impairment, although this is the ideal (Answers "a" and "d"). Clearly, the repair of a Concomitant Medical Condition does not signal the cure of Vince's diabetes (Answer "b"). The presence of a pathophysiological disorder (e.g., diabetes) does not automatically signal the presence of a Concomitant Medical Condition. Note that *all impairments—even Concomitant Medical Condition—refer to the behavioral/mental health aspects of patient dysfunction.*

4. Answer "a" is correct. Whereas goals always must be included in a discharge summary's PIP, the specific type of goal reported will depend on the overall objective of treatment. For Vince, all goals were identified as *endpoint* goals, based on the assumption that brief outpatient psychotherapy would be sufficient to treat his impairments. Other patients might have *interim, maintenance,* or *endpoint* goals, or a combination of all three, depending on the nature of treatment (see Chapter 5).

5. Answer "a" is correct. As stated above (see Answer 2), the presence of an impairment does not automatically imply the presence of a DSM-IV diagnosis (Answer "b"). It is true, however, that any significant patient dysfunction remaining at the time of treatment cessation should be reflected by an impairment in the discharge summary PIP with a severity rating of at least 1.

Epilogue

In this chapter, we briefly outline current developments regarding the Patient Impairment Profile (PIP) system, including software applications and future directions for research.

The PIP system offers a unique solution to the growing need for an inclusive nomenclature that addresses the question, Why is treatment needed? As such, it complements DSM-IV (American Psychiatric Association 1994), which addresses the important question, What is the diagnosis? Furthermore, the PIP system provides the means for establishing a comprehensive treatment database, a foundational prerequisite for the creation of valid practice guidelines for all mental health conditions. Given the initially promising research findings regarding the reliability and validity of the Impairment Lexicon, as documented by Klewicki et al. (1998) and Leucht et al. (1999), both of which are reprinted in Appendix B of this book, developing such a database appears increasingly feasible.

Practice Guidelines: A Win-Win-Win Scenario

In an era when many view managed care as advantageous for employers and managed care organizations (MCOs) but problematic for patients and practitioners, we envision uniform practice guidelines as an asset for all three groups. Clearly, such guidelines—when empirically supported by a large treatment database—will facilitate the efforts of MCOs to identify competent providers and appropriate treatment protocols, while guarding against unnecessary costs. Practitioners also will benefit because such guidelines will prevent third-party payers from inappropriately denying authorization for treatment when their own databases support such treatment protocols. Thus, we envision the stereotypically uniform authorization of four psychotherapy sessions—regardless of treatment needs—as a dinosaur whose extinction is imminent. Finally and most important, uniform practice guidelines would ensure that patients receive optimal care based on the collective findings of large treatment databases rather than on the individual opinion of one practitioner or one case reviewer. In short, uniform practice guidelines will facilitate the work of competent clinicians and help protect patients (and third-party payers) from those who are incompetent. At the same time, the collective wisdom of clinicians represented in treatment databases would help to keep the cost-cutting incentives of third-party payers in balance.

Some might argue that practice guidelines are too restrictive, but their benefits are already being recognized. For example, the American Psychiatric Association currently has developed such guidelines for ten major categories (e.g., schizophrenia, panic disorder, eating disorders) and made them available online (http://www.psych.org/clin_res/prac_guide.html); more are in development. Similarly, the Division of Clinical Psychology (Division 12) of the American Psychological Association has officially promoted the use of empirically validated treatment interventions since 1994. Specifically, Division 12 established an Implementation Committee for the Task Force on the Promotion and Dissemination of Psychological Procedures, and it has been publishing empirically supported psychological treatments since then (e.g., Sanderson 1994). Large-scale use of the PIP system could also provide the basis for empirically supported practice guidelines specific to impairments or patterns of impairments (PIPs). Such guidelines would focus primarily on patient goals and objectives, setting, length, and frequency and only secondarily on intervention types. Based on treatment outcome studies, these guidelines would increasingly emphasize empirically supported methods rather than professional guesswork.

The PIP and the Electronic Revolution

Managed care review based on telephone contact and/or use of paper reports and mail is quickly becoming obsolete. Not only are the costs of maintaining such bureaucracies prohibitive, but the time requirements for both practitioners and reviewers prevent cost-effective operation. In addition, the delays inherent in such procedures detract from optimal patient care. It is therefore not surprising that major third-party payers are converting to electronic information management systems. For example, since June 1996, Medicare in California has actively encouraged providers to convert to electronic claims processing methods, offering assistance to those willing to do so (Goodman et al. 1996). Clearly, survival in the burgeoning behavioral health marketplace will be more likely for those who can abandon paper and telephones in exchange for computers and modems. Indeed, because the current "handwriting on the wall" is electronic, only those who are computer literate will be able to read it.

The PIP system provides the means for successful transition. Preliminary research (Klewicki et al. 1998; Leucht et al. 1999; see Appendix B) suggests that—with appropriate training—practitioners can use the PIP system as a standardized method for treatment planning, documentation, and communication. Such a common language is crucial, particularly given the increasing prevalence of multidisciplinary treatment and the resulting need for continuity of information among practitioners from an array of disciplines and educational backgrounds.

The PIP is already being incorporated in a comprehensive software product. This product provides the means for accomplishing comprehensive, instant network communication among providers and those authorizing treatment. Automatic replication of relevant records eliminates the redundant characteristics of traditional documentation. In addition, those MCOs choosing to adopt this software as a communication standard for all providers will quickly generate clinically rich databases for measurement, assessment, and improvement of mental healthcare quality. Enhancements in quality measurement, empirical research, and general communication will be possible for both provider organizations and MCOs as a result of the common language furnished by the PIP system. Furthermore, information will be much more readily accessible and will also provide data for longitudinal studies of previously unobtainable magnitude. Studies using such software-generated data will be able to examine a multitude of potentially informative interrelationships, such as those between demographics, diagnoses, impairments, impairment severities, patient goals and objectives, interventions, treatment outcomes, and treatment settings, modalities, frequencies, and durations.

Current Research and Future Directions

As of the writing of this casebook, preliminary research findings regarding the PIP system have been favorable (Klewicki et al. 1998; Leucht et al. 1999; see Appendix B). These findings suggest that the Impairment Lexicon has promising reliability and validity, but the generalizability of these results is

Epilogue   **197**

limited. First, although the 20 patients depicted in these research studies (and presented in this case-book) portrayed every impairment included in the Impairment Lexicon, they represented only a small sampling of the diagnoses presented in DSM-IV.[1] Second, the extent to which ratings of vignettes generalize to ratings of actual patients is yet to be determined. Clearly, future research will need to assess the psychometric properties of the Impairment Lexicon when used to assess real persons seeking mental health services. Third, the raters in these preliminary studies were not mental health professionals but rather clinical psychology graduate students. Graduate students clearly have less clinical experience in assessing patients than do licensed mental health professionals, so this third methodological limitation actually might have reduced the strength of the findings. Thus, assessing the validity and reliability of the Impairment Lexicon with professional clinicians as raters might result in even more positive results.

Obviously, future research efforts should first address the methodological limitations of the preliminary studies. Thus, the reliability and validity of the Impairment Lexicon should be examined with patients manifesting a representative sample of DSM-IV diagnoses, and raters should be a representative sample of mental health professionals. Such psychometric research will be the basis for establishing the PIP system as a valid means of collecting clinical data.

The vast majority of meaningful and useful future research on the PIP system must extend beyond simple psychometric evaluations, however. Using computer technology to generate clinical treatment databases, researchers, in future studies, could address more central issues, such as treatment efficacy, cost-effectiveness, recidivism, and practice guidelines for individual impairments and impairment constellations. Our vision is that such research would contribute to a greater understanding of behavioral health concerns, facilitate the optimizing of effective treatment models, and provide an ongoing basis for the continued improvement of patient care. Even in an increasingly cost-conscious environment, such factors deserve the primary ongoing attention of all those invested in the healing vocations.

---

[1]The 20 vignettes presented in this book contain minor stylistic modifications, but they are essentially identical to those used in the research.

Appendix A

DSM-IV Diagnostic Criteria for the Vignette Patients

Note to the reader: *For each vignette patient, the specific DSM-IV (American Psychiatric Association 1994) diagnostic criteria are summarized. Supportive evidence for criteria is presented in italic type.*

Case Presentation 1: "Frank"

DSM-IV Axis I diagnosis: 295.30 Schizophrenia, paranoid type

DSM-IV criteria for schizophrenia

A. Psychotic symptoms for 1 or more weeks (*Frank reports hallucinations and bizarre delusions.*)

B. Functioning markedly impaired relative to highest level achieved before onset of schizophrenia (*Frank obtained a high school diploma.*)

C. Continuous signs of disturbance for 6 months or more (*Frank has received psychiatric medication continuously since age 18.*)

D. Not due to schizoaffective disorder or mood disorder with psychotic features

E. Not due to the effects of a substance (medication, abused drug) or a medical condition (*Frank is not abusing any substances.*)

F. No history of a pervasive developmental disorder

DSM-IV criteria for paranoid subtype

A. Preoccupation with one or more delusions or auditory hallucinations (*Frank has demonstrated both.*)

B. None of the following prominent: disorganized speech, disorganized or catatonic behavior, or flat or inappropriate affect

DSM-IV Axis II diagnosis: None

199

Case Presentation 2: "Shirley"

DSM-IV Axis I diagnosis: 300.3 Obsessive-compulsive disorder

DSM-IV criteria for obsessive-compulsive disorder

A. Either obsessions or compulsions:

   Obsessions (*Shirley meets all four criteria for obsessions.*)

   Compulsions (*Shirley meets all four criteria for compulsions.*)

B. Recognizes that obsessions and compulsions are excessive and unreasonable (*Shirley admits, "I know it's crazy."*)

C. The obsessions and compulsions cause marked distress and are time-consuming (*Shirley's obsessions/compulsions occur multiple times per day; her hand-washing consumes 1 hour or more per day.*)

D. No other Axis I disorder is present

E. Not due to the effects of a substance (medication, abused drug) or a medical condition (*Shirley is not abusing any substances.*)

DSM-IV Axis II diagnosis: None

Case Presentation 3: "Yolanda"

DSM-IV Axis I diagnosis: 305.00 Alcohol abuse

DSM-IV criteria for alcohol abuse

A. Evidence of a maladaptive pattern of use leading to clinically significant impairment or distress within 12 months, as manifested by one or more of four criteria (*Yolanda's behavior meets the first two criteria.*)

   Criterion 1 (*Yolanda's substance abuse is resulting in failure to meet expectations at work and difficulties concentrating.*)

   Criterion 2 (*Yolanda's abuse also occurs while operating heavy machinery.*)

B. Symptoms have never met criteria for alcohol dependence (*This is Yolanda's first bout of abuse.*)

DSM-IV Axis II diagnosis: None

Appendix A: DSM-IV Diagnostic Criteria for Vignette Patients

Case Presentation 4: "Pam"

DSM-IV Axis I diagnosis: 307.51 Bulimia nervosa

DSM-IV criteria for bulimia nervosa

A. Recurrent uncontrolled binges (*Pam reports eating "lots of junk food...once or twice a week." She further states that "once I started eating, I couldn't stop."*)

B. Recurrent inappropriate compensatory behavior (*Pam vomits regularly.*)

C. Two or more binge and purge episodes per week for 3 months (*Pam's episodes began 8 months ago.*)

D. Self-evaluation unduly influenced by body shape and weight (*Pam's reason for her suicidal gesture is "I'm tired of being so fat."*)

E. Disturbance does not occur exclusively during episodes of anorexia nervosa

DSM-IV Axis II diagnosis: None

Case Presentation 5: "George"

DSM-IV Axis I diagnosis: 302.2 Pedophilia, sexually attracted to both

DSM-IV criteria for pedophilia, sexually attracted to both

A. Disturbance of at least 6 months; recurrent sexual urges and fantasies involving sexual activity with a prepubescent child (*George has been sexually abusing his daughter during the past year, and he allegedly abused his son several years ago.*)

B. The sexual urges and behaviors have caused clinically significant impairment in social functioning (*George's behavior has negatively affected the social functioning of his family.*)

C. The individual is older than 16 years and is at least 5 years older than the child (*George is 40, and Samantha is 10.*)

DSM-IV Axis II diagnosis: None

Case Presentation 6: "Mark"

DSM-IV Axis I diagnosis: 302.85 Gender identity disorder

DSM-IV criteria for gender identity disorder

A. A strong and persistent cross-gender identification, manifested by a stated desire to be the opposite gender (*Mark wishes "to be a woman."*)

B. Persistent discomfort with his or her sex and gender role (*Mark is "tired of being a man" and "want[s] a sex change operation."*)

C. The disturbance is not concurrent with a physical intersex condition

D. The disturbance causes clinically significant distress in social functioning (*Mark and his spouse are experiencing marital distress.*)

DSM-IV Axis II diagnosis: None

Case Presentation 7: "Tamara"

DSM-IV Axis I diagnosis: 300.14 Dissociative identity disorder

DSM-IV criteria for dissociative identity disorder

A. Presence of two or more distinct identities or personality states (*Tamara identifies herself as "Angel" and does not remember doing so later.*)

B. Two or more of these identities or personality states recurrently take full control of the person's behavior (*"Angel" burns herself.*)

C. Inability to recall important personal information not due to ordinary forgetfulness (*Tamara has no recollection of "Angel" and vice versa.*)

D. Disturbance is not due to the effects of a substance (medication, abused drug) or a medical condition (*Tamara is not abusing any substance.*)

DSM-IV Axis II diagnosis: None

Appendix A: DSM-IV Diagnostic Criteria for Vignette Patients   **203**

Case Presentation 8: "Juan"

DSM-IV Axis I diagnosis: 309.81 Posttraumatic stress disorder

DSM-IV criteria for posttraumatic stress disorder

A. Exposure to a traumatic event in which the following were present:

(1) experience of a threat to physical integrity of self (*Juan was sexually molested.*)

(2) intense fear response and/or (in children) agitated behavior (*Juan screams on waking at night. In session, he bangs toys together when asked about the event.*)

B. Traumatic event persistently reexperienced (*Juan has engaged in reenactive sexual play, has nightmares, and shows distress when the event is simply mentioned [e.g., bangs toys together].*)

C. Persistent avoidance of trauma-associated stimuli (*Juan refuses to discuss the event; he states, "Don't let him come over anymore, Mommy!"; and he shows a restricted range of affect by being less affectionate.*)

D. Persistent increased arousal (*Juan has trouble falling asleep and is generally irritable.*)

E. Duration of symptoms for more than 1 month (*Juan's symptoms have been present for 7 weeks so far.*)

F. Disturbance causes clinically significant distress or impairment in school functioning (*Juan insisted that other children "play doctor" at school.*)

DSM-IV Axis II diagnosis: None

Case Presentation 9: "Wanda"

DSM-IV Axis I diagnosis: 296.22 Major depression, single episode, moderate

DSM-IV criteria for 296.22 major depression, single episode, moderate

A. Single major depressive episode, moderate[a]

   (1) Five or more symptoms of the nine listed in DSM-IV (*Wanda has depressed mood, diminished interest, decreased appetite, fatigue, and recurrent thoughts about her grandmother's death.*)

   (2) Does not meet mixed episode criteria

   (3) Symptoms cause clinically significant distress or impairment

   (4) Not due to the effects of a substance or medical condition

   (5) Not due to normal bereavement (*Wanda did not know her grandmother very well; her grandmother lived 2,000 miles away.*)

B. Not part of a schizoaffective disorder or superimposed on a thought disorder

C. No manic/hypomanic history

Note. [a]Wanda's major depression is moderate because it has affected school attendance but not performance yet.

DSM-IV Axis II diagnosis: None

Case Presentation 10: "Carlos"

DSM-IV Axis I diagnosis: None

DSM-IV criteria for antisocial personality disorder

A. Evidence of antisocial behavior since age 15, as indicated by three or more of the seven symptoms listed in DSM-IV (*Carlos has been arrested frequently, has shown impulsivity, has a history of physical fights, has never held a steady job, and shows no remorse for his actions.*)

B. Age 18 or older (*Carlos is 41.*)

C. Evidence of conduct disorder before age 15 with 3 or more of the 15 symptoms listed in DSM-IV (*Carlos often started fights, stole things, and was truant.*)

D. Does not occur during mania or schizophrenia

DSM-IV Axis II diagnosis: 301.7 Antisocial personality disorder

Appendix A: DSM-IV Diagnostic Criteria for Vignette Patients

Case Presentation 11: "April"

DSM-IV Axis I diagnosis: 295.10 Schizophrenia, disorganized type

DSM-IV criteria for schizophrenia

A. Psychotic symptoms for 1 or more weeks (*April has bizarre delusions, incoherence, and flat affect.*)

B. Functioning markedly impaired relative to highest level achieved before onset (*April had been staying in her own semi-independent apartment.*)

C. Continuous signs of disturbance for 6 or more months

D. Not due to schizoaffective disorder or mood disorder with psychotic features

E. Not due to the effects of a substance (medication, abused drug) or a medical condition

F. No history of a pervasive developmental disorder

DSM-IV criteria for disorganized subtype

A. Disorganized speech and behavior; or inappropriate affect (*April has demonstrated both.*)

B. Does not meet criteria for catatonic type

DSM-IV Axis II diagnosis: None

Case Presentation 12: "Billy"

DSM-IV Axis I diagnosis: 307.6 Enuresis, nocturnal only

DSM-IV criteria for enuresis, nocturnal only

A. Repeated involuntary or intentional voiding of urine into bed or clothes

B. Two or more events per week for 3 or more months (*Billy has never achieved full nocturnal bladder control.*)

C. Chronological age of 5 or older (or equivalent developmental level)

D. Not due to the effects of a substance (medication, abused drug) or a medical condition

DSM-IV Axis II diagnosis: None

Case Presentation 13: "Hannah"

DSM-IV Axis I diagnosis: 314.01 Attention-deficit/hyperactivity disorder

DSM-IV criteria for attention-deficit/hyperactivity disorder

A. Either Criterion 1 or Criterion 2 *(Hannah meets Criterion 2.)*

Criterion 2: Disturbance for 6 or more months, with six or more of the nine symptoms listed in DSM-IV *(For the past 3 years, Hannah often fidgets, leaves her seat, is constantly "on the go," has difficulty playing quietly, talks excessively, blurts out answers, and interrupts others.)*

B. Onset before age 7 years *(Hannah's symptoms were apparent at age 6.)*

C. Some impairment from symptoms present in two or more settings *(Hannah has similar problems both at school and at home.)*

D. Evidence of clinically significant impairment in social and academic functioning *(Hannah has a mathematics disorder and behavior problems at school and at home.)*

E. Symptoms are not better accounted for by another mental disorder (e.g., pervasive developmental disorder, thought disorder, mood disorder)

DSM-IV Axis I *dual* diagnosis: 307.7 Encopresis

DSM-IV criteria for encopresis

A. Repeated passage of feces into inappropriate places *(Hannah soils her clothing.)*

B. One or more events per month for at least 3 months *(Hannah soils once per month.)*

C. Chronological age of 4 or older (or equivalent developmental level)

D. Not due to the effects of a substance (medication, abused drug) or a medical condition

DSM-IV Axis I *dual* diagnosis: 315.1 Mathematics disorder

DSM-IV criteria for mathematics disorder

A. Standardized tests indicate that arithmetic skills are markedly below the expected level given age, educational level, and overall measured intelligence *(Hannah's test results meet these criteria.)*

B. This disturbance in Criterion A significantly interferes with academic achievement *(Hannah is receiving poor math grades.)*

C. Not due to a sensory deficit if one is present *(None is present.)*

DSM-IV Axis II diagnosis: None

Appendix A: DSM-IV Diagnostic Criteria for Vignette Patients **207**

Case Presentation 14: "Zack"

DSM-IV Axis I diagnosis: 312.31 Pathological gambling

DSM-IV criteria for pathological gambling

A. Persistent and recurrent maladaptive gambling behavior as indicated by the presence of 5 or more of the 10 symptoms listed in DSM-IV (*Zack is preoccupied with gambling, must risk higher amounts to achieve the desired excitement, tries to "chase" his losses, is jeopardizing his marriage, and is using his wife's salary to support his gambling.*)

B. Not due to a manic episode

DSM-IV Axis II diagnosis: V71.09 None, narcissistic traits

DSM-IV criteria for narcissistic traits

A. Symptomatology is not sufficient for the diagnosis of 301.81 narcissistic personality disorder

B. Some traits associated with narcissistic personality disorder are present (*Zack has a grandiose self-image, exploits others for his advantage, and lacks empathy.*)

Case Presentation 15: "Dean"

DSM-IV Axis I diagnosis: 296.03 Bipolar I disorder, single manic episode

DSM-IV criteria for bipolar I disorder, single manic episode

A. Currently in a manic episode

(1) A distinct period of abnormally and persistently elevated, expansive, or irritated mood, involving hospitalization

(2) Three or more of the seven symptoms listed in DSM-IV (*Dean has shown a decreased need for sleep, pressured speech, and increased goal-directed activity in his small business, and he has gone on buying sprees.*)

(3) Symptoms do not meet criteria for a mixed episode

(4) Mood disturbance causes marked impairment in occupational and social functioning (*Dean's co-workers have complained about his being too intense.*)

(5) Not due to the effects of a substance (medication, abused drug) or medical condition (*Dean has not been using any substances or medications.*)

B. Presence of only one manic episode and no past major depressive episodes (*No other episodes have been documented.*)

C. Not part of a schizoaffective disorder or superimposed on a thought disorder

DSM-IV Axis II diagnosis: None

Appendix A: DSM-IV Diagnostic Criteria for Vignette Patients   **209**

Case Presentation 16: "Lilly"

DSM-IV Axis I diagnosis: 300.4 Dysthymic disorder

DSM-IV criteria for dysthymic disorder

A. Predominantly depressed mood for at least 2 years (*Lilly has been "always down" for at least the last 2 years.*)

B. While depressed, more than two of the 6 symptoms listed in DSM-IV are present (*Lilly has been overeating and complains of constant fatigue.*)

C. During the past 2 years, symptoms have never failed to meet Criteria A and B for more than 2 months (*Lilly's symptoms have been continuous.*)

D. Not due to a major depressive disorder

E. No history of hypomanic, manic, or mixed episode or cyclothymic disorder

F. Not due to a chronic psychotic disorder

G. Not due to the effects of a substance (medication, abused drug) or medical condition (*Lilly is not using any substances or medications.*)

H. Symptoms cause clinically significant social distress or impairment (*Lilly sought services because of marital problems related to her symptomatology.*)

DSM-IV Axis II diagnosis: 301.50 Histrionic personality disorder

DSM-IV criteria for histrionic personality disorder

A. A histrionic pattern of behavior, as indicated by five or more of the eight symptoms listed in DSM-IV (*Lilly shows seductive behavior even in the interview, her emotions rapidly shift, she dresses provocatively "whenever she goes out," her speech lacks detail, and her emotional expression is theatrically exaggerated.*)

Case Presentation 17: "Eddie"

DSM-IV Axis I diagnosis: 309.21 Separation anxiety disorder

DSM-IV criteria for separation anxiety disorder

A. Expresses excessive separation anxiety, as shown by three or more of the eight symptoms listed in DSM-IV (*Eddie becomes overly distressed whenever he is apart from his mother, expresses fear that his mother will not come back whenever she leaves him, refuses to go to school, and complains of stomachaches and headaches.*)

B. The disturbance has lasted 4 or more weeks (*Eddie's symptoms have been present for 3 months.*)

C. Onset is before age 18 years

D. The disturbance causes clinically significant distress and impairment in social and academic functioning (*Eddie's school attendance has been poor, and he has had frequent temper tantrums.*)

E. Not due to pervasive developmental disorder, schizophrenia, or other psychotic disorder

DSM-IV Axis II diagnosis: None

Case Presentation 18: "Karen"

DSM-IV Axis I diagnosis: 313.81 Oppositional defiant disorder

DSM-IV criteria for oppositional defiant disorder

A. A pattern of negativistic, hostile, and defiant behavior for 6 or more months, evidenced by four or more of the eight symptoms listed in DSM-IV (*Karen frequently loses her temper, argues with adults, defies her mother's rules, and seems easily annoyed, quite resentful, and angry.*)

B. Behavior disturbance has caused clinically significant distress and impairment in social functioning (*Karen's behavior is contributing to distress and dysfunction within her family.*)

C. Not due to a psychotic or mood disorder

D. Not due to a conduct disorder

DSM-IV Axis II diagnosis: None

Appendix A: DSM-IV Diagnostic Criteria for Vignette Patients **211**

Case Presentation 19: "Inez"

DSM-IV Axis I diagnosis: 300.29 Specific phobia

DSM-IV criteria for specific phobia

A. Marked and persistent unreasonable fear of a specific object (*Inez fears dogs, specifically fearing that they will attack her.*)

B. Exposure to the specific phobic stimulus almost invariably provokes an immediate anxiety response (*When Inez sees or hears a dog—even on TV—it results in a fear response, such as racing pulse.*)

C. The person recognizes that the fear is excessive or unreasonable (*Inez describes her fear as "crazy," and "silly."*)

D. The object or situation is avoided (*Inez avoids the park where she saw a dog bite a young girl; she rarely goes outside the home without her husband.*)

E. The fear of the avoidant behavior significantly interferes with the person's usual social activities and relationships with others (*Inez does not feel comfortable going out with friends; she is too embarrassed to talk with friends on the telephone.*)

F. In persons younger than 18 years, symptoms have persisted for more than 6 months (*Inez is older than 18.*)

G. The phobia is not related to another disorder (e.g., obsessive-compulsive disorder, posttraumatic stress disorder, panic disorder with agoraphobia)

DSM-IV Axis II diagnosis: None

Case Presentation 20: "Vince"

DSM-IV Axis I diagnosis: 296.21 Major depression, single episode, mild

DSM-IV criteria for major depression, single episode, mild

A. Single major depressive episode, mild[a]

   (1) Five or more of the nine symptoms listed in DSM-IV (*Vince has reported depressed mood, weight gain, insomnia, fatigue, and recurrent thoughts of death.*)

   (2) Does not meet mixed episode criteria

   (3) Symptoms cause clinically significant distress or impairment

   (4) Not due to the effects of a substance (medication, abused drug) or medical condition (*Vince's medical condition is related to, but not the cause of, his depression.*)

   (5) Not due to *normal* bereavement

B. Not part of a schizoaffective disorder or superimposed on a thought disorder

C. No manic or hypomanic history

Note. [a]Symptoms do not exceed those needed for diagnosis and cause only minor impairment in usual activities.

DSM-IV Axis II diagnosis: None

Appendix B

Empirical Research Articles

Psychological Reports, 1998, 83, 547-570. © Psychological Reports 1998

PATIENT IMPAIRMENT LEXICON: A PSYCHOMETRIC ANALYSIS[1]

LISA L. KLEWICKI, JEFFREY P. BJORCK, CHRISTOPHER A. LEUCHT

Graduate School of Psychology
Fuller Theological Seminary

MICHAEL GOODMAN

UCLA School of Medicine
Department of Psychiatry and Biobehavioral Sciences

Summary.—Growth in managed care has magnified the needs for assessment of treatment efficacies and standardized communication regarding treatment needs. Addressing both needs requires a common terminology describing the scope of treatable mental health impairments. The Diagnostic and Statistical Manual of Mental Disorders-IV provides a common categorical language for describing clinical disorders, but its categories are not discrete and do little to facilitate communication regarding specific treatment needs. Goodman, Brown, and Deitz developed a Patient Impairment Lexicon intended to address these limitations. The current vignette study provided initial psychometric assessment of this nomenclature, specifically examining interrater reliability, temporal stability, and content validity. Findings are discussed with respect to both applications in managed care and psychometric research.

Managed care's influence on mental health treatment is steadily increasing, with as many of 75% of clinical psychologists reporting some level of participation as providers (Norcross, Karg, & Prochaska, 1997). Currently, managed care networks reimburse treatment providers based upon specifically identified disorders (Taube, Lee, & Forthofer, 1984) and their corresponding "accepted" treatment (Barlow, 1994). Increasingly, however, treatment efficacy and cost efficiency are being emphasized as primary bases for reimbursement (Barlow, 1994). In order to assess treatment efficacy empirically, a common and universal nomenclature for treatable impairments is needed to facilitate communication and generalization of findings regarding treatment efficacy for specific mental health impairments.

The Diagnostic and Statistical Manual of Mental Disorders-IV (American Psychiatric Association, 1994) provides a nomenclature for identifying disorders, not only for psychologists and psychiatrists but for all mental health professionals and medical personnel. Revisions of this diagnostic lan-

---

[1]This article is based on a dissertation completed by Lisa L. Klewicki under the direction of Jeffrey P. Bjorck at the Graduate School of Psychology, Fuller Theological Seminary. Thanks go to Richard L. Gorsuch and Stephen N. Haynes for providing helpful feedback on an earlier version of this article. Send correspondence to Jeffrey P. Bjorck, Graduate School of Psychology, Fuller Theological Seminary, 180 North Oakland Avenue, Pasadena, California 91101.

Reproduced with permission of the authors and publisher from:

Klewicki L. L., Bjorck J. P., & Leucht C. A.: Patient Impairment Lexicon: A Psychometric Analysis. *Psychological Reports* 83:547–570, 1998. Copyright © 1998 Psychological Reports.

guage have been increasingly empirically based, from the theoretically based first edition of the DSM (American Psychiatric Association, 1952) to the current form which "more than any other nomenclature of mental disorders . . . is grounded in empirical evidence" (p. xvi).

Although the DSM-IV represents the most empirically based system of diagnostic classifications it still has some limitations regarding goals and the extent to which these are accomplished. For example, the DSM-IV is designed to "divide mental disorders into types based on criteria sets with defining features" (p. xxii). The authors acknowledge, however, that the categorical approach to diagnosing mental disorders does not provide completely discrete diagnostic categories and individuals "sharing a diagnosis are likely to be heterogeneous even in regard to the defining features of the diagnosis" (p. xxii). Thus, the resulting overlap of categories and variance within each category weakens the reliability and validity of the system (e.g., Clark, Watson, & Reynolds, 1995; Hayes, Wilson, Gifford, Follette, & Strosahl, 1996; Lilienfeld, Waldman, & Israel, 1994; Widiger & Ford-Black, 1994; Wulfert, Greenway, & Dougher, 1996). Given these weaknesses, Calhoun, Moras, Pilkonis, and Rehm (1998) recommend that DSM-IV should not be the sole criteria for treatment decisions. Similarly, Goldfried and Wolfe (1998) propose that research regarding treatment outcome should increasingly use "methodology that emphasizes greater homogeneity of clinical problems" (p. 148).

In addition, the DSM-IV has limited utility regarding development of treatment plans. To its credit, the manual acknowledges that diagnosis is only a "first step in a comprehensive evaluation . . . [and that] . . . the clinician will invariably require considerable additional information about the person being evaluated" to develop an adequate treatment plan (DSM-IV, p. xxv). As managed care networks have increasingly required practitioners to document justifiable treatment plans, the need for such information has increased. Indeed, in response to the need for efficient and effective treatment, many managed care organizations have developed their own idiosyncratic supplementary rating systems as a basis for determining the extent of reimbursement. Thus, in addition to requiring clinicians provide DSM-IV diagnoses, many managed care organizations require them to state why the patient needs treatment.[2] Clinicians' unstandardized responses are then used as a major factor in determining reimbursement (Goodman, Brown, & Deitz, 1996).

The need for standardized nomenclature to address the question, "Why

---

[2]The word "patient" is used in the current study as a general reference to someone using mental health services, regardless of setting. Thus, "patients" could also be referred to as "clients" in some settings, e.g., outpatient.

Appendix B: Empirical Research Articles

PATIENT IMPAIRMENT LEXICON

is treatment needed?" is readily apparent. For example, whereas ten patients on a psychiatric unit might all be diagnosed with "major depression," each one might present with different impairments representing unique treatment needs. To address this issue, Goodman, Brown, & Deitz (1992) proposed a common nomenclature of behavioral impairments, each representing a potential reason for mental health treatment. Their Patient Impairment Lexicon originally included 65 operationally defined impairments, intended as a comprehensive list of potential foci for mental health treatment. Revision of the Patient Impairment Lexicon resulted in a lexicon containing 63 such terms (Goodman, *et al.*, 1996; Haynes, Richard, & Kubany, 1995).

The Patient Impairment Lexicon is used to create a Patient Impairment Profile for a given patient. The profile lists those impairments identified as treatment foci, together with a severity rating for each, i.e., 1 = "distressing," 2 = "destabilizing," 3 = "incapacitating," 4 = "imminently dangerous." Impairment presentation in the profile is prioritized according to the clinician's judgments regarding severity. It is important to note that these severity ratings indicate the extent to which each impairment compromises the patient's normal functioning, not how upsetting a given impairment is for the patient. The profile identifies behavioral impairments, thus augmenting DSM-IV diagnostic information by communicating specific treatment needs to reviewers. Also, the profile facilitates treatment planning because the prioritized impairments listed there logically imply specific prioritized goals for treatment, i.e., the repair or reduction to maintenance level of each identified impairment. These goals, in turn, provide a basis for the selection of treatment objectives and interventions. Furthermore, the profile is designed to document patients' progress over time via the ratings of severity of impairment.

The Patient Impairment Lexicon addresses the limitations of DSM-IV's categorical diagnostic nomenclature in two ways. First, in the former, impairments are intended to be specific and mutually exclusive; each impairment describes a discrete observable constellation of behavior and is designed to have no overlap with other impairments. For example, Altered Sleep is defined as "any disruption of the normal 24-hour sleep-wake cycle, including insomnia, hypersomnia, early morning awakening, or night terrors (Goodman, *et al.*, 1996, p. 171). Given this greater specificity and exclusivity, the behaviors attributed to a given impairment are more homogeneous than those included within a given DSM-IV diagnostic category.

Second, the Patient Impairment Profile provides quantitative ratings of judged severity for each impairment. In contrast, although the DSM-IV acknowledges the benefits of classifying "clinical presentations based on quantification of attributes rather than assignment to categories" (p. xxii), it maintains a solely categorical approach. Quantitative judgments, however, can provide higher reliability than categorical ones. For example, Heumann and

550   L. L. KLEWICKI, *ET AL.*

Morey (1990) asked five mental health professionals (psychiatrists and psychologists) to rate 10 case vignettes as to whether the patient depicted in the vignette met the Diagnostic and Statistical Manual of Mental Disorders-III, revised (American Psychiatric Association, 1987) criteria for a personality disorder, i.e., a categorical judgment and also to assess the same vignette using four different behavioral scales. All four of these quantitative judgments provided greater reliability estimates than the categorical DSM-III–R diagnosis.

The criteria for psychometrically evaluating a diagnostic system are often quantifiable observable behaviors (e.g., Atrom, Thorell, Homlund, & d'Elia, 1993; Coleman, Carpener, Waternaux, Levy, Shenton, Perry, Medoff, Wong, Monoach, Meyer, O'Brian, Valentino, Robinson, Smith, Makowski, & Holzman, 1993; Evenson & Boyd, 1993; Kaplan, 1993; Ponsford & Kinsella, 1991). The behavioral specificity inherent in the lexicon should facilitate its psychometric evaluation. If shown to be reliable and valid, the lexicon could facilitate the ongoing empirical efforts to evaluate relationships between patients' dysfunctions, modalities of intervention, and efficacy of treatment. Specifically, if used as a "single standard measure" (p. 1070, Sechrest, McKnight, & McKnight, 1996) for classifying patients' impairments, the Patient Impairment Lexicon could readily be used to generate reliable research data. There would also be practical advantages of using the lexicon to identify treatable behavioral impairments. First, the lexicon provides a common nomenclature of observable behavior, readily understandable by all persons involved, e.g., mental health professionals, case managers, managed care reviewers. Goodman, *et al.* (1996) state, "Impairments are 'behavioral windows' into the aberrant biochemical phenomena and psychological variations of existence that are the etiology of psychiatric disorders" (p. 29). As such, the lexicon could provide a basis for standardized documentation (Chrisman, Lancaster, Ross, Ainsworth, Hemmings, & Shaffer, 1996). Second, the behavioral emphasis of the lexicon's impairment definitions could provide a basis for treatment planning and managed care decisions regarding reimbursement.

As a preliminary psychometric evaluation, we assessed the interrater reliability of the lexicon and its temporal stability and content validity. Evaluating the entire lexicon requires that it be applied to cases manifesting all 63 impairments. This was done by carefully constructing 20 vignettes, each depicting one prototypical patient such that the 20 patients collectively represented the Patient Impairment Lexicon's entire range of impairments.

Lanza and Carifio (1992) discussed the methodological advantages of vignettes. For example, using the same vignettes across different raters enables methodological standardization. Several psychometric studies of diagnostic systems have used case vignettes in this way (e.g., Andersen & Harthorn, 1989; Hasin & Link, 1988; Heumann & Morey, 1990; Hjortso, But-

Appendix B: Empirical Research Articles

PATIENT IMPAIRMENT LEXICON

ler, Clemmensen, Jepsen, Kastrup, Vilmar, & Bech, 1989; Marwit, 1996; Sorensen, Hargreaves, & Friedlander, 1982; Shepherd, Brooke, Cooper, & Lin, 1968). Moreover, material observed or read in case vignettes remains constant across raters, facilitating assessment of interrater reliability (Hjortso, *et al.*, 1989). Vignettes also facilitate assessment of temporal stability because the described patients remain constant over time. If vignette studies support the Patient Impairment Lexicon's utility, it will then be appropriate to examine its application to actual cases. Given the low incidence of some patient dysfunctions, however, this would require hundreds—if not thousands—of patients to ensure sufficient data to test all 63 impairments. Thus, whereas vignettes obviously limit generalizability of findings, their use represents a cost-effective primary evaluation of a classification system (Hjortso, *et al,* 1989; Marwit, 1996).

Given that documentation of patients' impairments involves multiple raters, the need to evaluate the interrater reliability of the lexicon is clear. High interrater agreement is a prerequisite for any nomenclature intended to provide standardized communication (Nunnally & Bernstein, 1994). In contrast, such a nomenclature would not typically be expected to have high test-retest reliability, given that mental health impairments change over time. Vignettes of "patients," however, do not change over time. Thus, given a sufficient interval to address memory effects, temporal stability assessment of ratings of vignette "patients" can provide another estimate of the lexicon's reliability.

Once the reliability of a measure is supported, content validity can be a first step in the process of construct validation. Haynes, *et al.* (1995) define content validity as "the degree to which elements of an assessment instrument are relevant to and representative of the targeted construct for a particular assessment purpose" (p. 238). The lexicon's targeted construct is treatable mental health impairments, and its assessment purpose is to answer the diagnostic question of "Why does the patient need treatment?" Thus, to exhibit optimal content validity, the 63 impairments in the Patient Impairment Lexicon should represent the entire domain of potential reasons for mental health treatment, with no overlap of items. With these goals in mind, recent content revisions of the lexicon (Goodman, *et al.*, 1996) were made to improve both the inclusivity and exclusivity of each of the 63 impairments. These revisions were based on a series of qualitative examinations culminating in 100% consensus of all four authors. Using this revised lexicon, the current study further evaluated content validity by examining the accuracy, specificity, and clarity of the lexicon's 63 items (Haynes, *et al.*, 1995).

In summary, the current study is a psychometric evaluation of the Patient Impairment Lexicon using case vignettes to facilitate methodological standardization and evaluation of interrater reliability and temporal stability.

552   L. L. KLEWICKI, *ET AL.*

We hypothesized the clinicians rating case vignettes would agree in their use of the entire lexicon, as evidenced by high interrater reliability and temporal stability across all 63 impairments. We further hypothesized that raters would agree in their use of each individual term describing an impairment. We also examined the content validity. First, the examination of interrater agreement regarding individual impairments served as a quantitative measure of rater accuracy and specificity, relative to the intended depictions of impairments. Second, we qualitatively assessed the extent to which the lexicon depicts the entire domain of treatable mental health impairments by asking raters to offer suggestions for additional impairments. We hypothesized that raters would propose no additions to the lexicon.

METHOD

Measures

Impairment Inventory.—To facilitate evaluation of the lexicon, an Impairment Inventory was constructed, presenting Goodman, *et al.*'s (1996) 63 impairment terms alphabetically (without definitions) in two columns on an $8^{1}/_{2}$- × 11-in. sheet. Adjacent to each impairment term is Goodman, *et al.*'s 4-point severity scale, i.e., 1 = distressing: causing mental anguish or suffering in self/others; 2 = destabilizing: markedly weakens the ability to carry out daily activities and/or places self/others in potential danger; 3 = incapacitating: severely interferes with normal daily functioning and/or places self/others in likely danger; 4 = imminently dangerous: immediately life-threatening to self/others. An Impairment Inventory is used for each identified patient. Specifically, raters circle impairment terms that they believe describe the patient's functioning and then rate the severity of each circled impairment on its adjacent 4-point scale. Impairments not circled were assigned a severity rating of zero.

Vignettes.—Twenty vignettes depicted descriptions of 20 patients (5–73 yr. old; $M = 26.75$), each being seen for an initial clinical interview. Each vignette was approximately one page in length and presented (a) reasons for referral, (b) relevant history, (c) clinical presentation, and (d) assumptions about the assessment, e.g., that symptoms were not organic. The vignettes were equally divided into five commonly identified case types: (a) chronic adult, (b) acute adult, (c) child, (d) family, and (e) couple. Each identified patient met the criteria for a DSM-III–R diagnosis (see Table 1). The DSM-III–R disorders and diagnostic criteria were used in order to compare the Patient Impairment Lexicon to a well established diagnostic system familiar to raters (the DSM-IV was only recently in print when data were collected). The 20 descriptions served as "subjects" (see Appendix for an example vignette, pp. 569-570).

Each of the 63 impairments from the lexicon was depicted within at

Appendix B: Empirical Research Articles

TABLE 1
CHARACTERISTICS OF VIGNETTES

Vignette	Age	Sex	Ethnicity	Diagnosis (DSM-III-R)	Type of Case
1	35	Female	Asian American	Schizophrenia, disorganized	Chronic adult
2	24	Male	Euro-American	Schizophrenia, paranoid	Chronic adult
3	41	Male	Latino	Antisocial personality disorder	Chronic adult
4	21	Female	African American	Multiple personality disorder	Chronic adult
5	73	Male	African American	Major depression, single, mild	Nonchronic adult
6	32	Male	Euro-American	Bipolar, manic	Nonchronic adult
7	47	Female	African American	Obsessive-compulsive disorder	Nonchronic adult
8	24	Female	Latina	Alcohol abuse	Nonchronic adult
9	7	Male	Latino	Post-traumatic stress disorder	Child
10	5	Male	African American	Functional enuresis, primary	Child
11	9	Female	Euro-American	Attention deficit/hyperactivity disorder, functional encopresis	Child
12	15	Female	Euro-American	Bulimia nervosa	Child
13	40	Male	African American	Pedophilia	Family
14	8	Male	Latino	Separation anxiety	Family
15	14	Female	African American	Major depression, single, moderate	Family
16	16	Female	Asian American	Oppositional defiant disorder	Family
17	30	Male	Euro-American	Pathological gambling	Couple
18	37	Female	Latina	Simple phobia	Couple
19	28	Female	Asian American	Dysthymia, histrionic personality disorder	Couple
20	29	Male	Asian American	Male erectile disorder	Couple

least one of the 20 vignettes. Seven of the 63 impairments were depicted in more than one vignette in order for the identified patient to meet a DSM-III–R diagnosis.[3] As part of vignette construction (Heverly, Fitt, & Newman, 1984; Lanza & Carifio, 1992), content validity of the 20 vignettes was maximized through a series of collective revisions by a psychiatrist, a psychologist, and two doctoral students in clinical psychology. Revisions involved assessing each vignette in terms of (a) face validity, (b) inclusion of intended impairments, (c) exclusion of unintended impairments, and (d) inclusion of sufficient criteria for DSM-III–R diagnosis. The identified patient within each vignette met the criteria for at least one DSM-III–R diagnosis. A wide range of diagnoses was presented (see Table 1). Furthermore, the identified patients across the 20 vignettes equally represented both sexes and four ethnic groups (i.e., Euro-American, Latino, African American, and Asian American; see Table 1).

Procedure

Sixteen graduate students (4th, 5th, or 6th year) from a doctoral program in southern California in clinical psychology served as raters of the 20 patients described in the vignettes. Raters were paid for participating and were initially presented the measures via group administration. Prior to completing the measures, raters were provided with detailed written instructions, an example vignette, and corresponding examples of completed measures. Aside from these instructions, raters received no training. To minimize confounding variables, instructions included the assumption that all identified patients were fully fluent in English and completely acculturated to life within the United States. (Whereas ethnocultural variables merit direct investigation, they were beyond the current study's scope.)

Next, all materials were provided to each rater in a booklet including the 20 vignettes in counterbalanced order and 20 corresponding Impairment Inventories. Raters also received two reference sheets listing the Patient Impairment Lexicon's impairment definitions and the rating scale for severity (Goodman, *et al.*, 1996), respectively. Raters were instructed to imagine that they were conducting the clinical interviews depicted in the vignettes. Any

---

[3] Altered Sleep, Egocentricity, and Inadequate Self-maintenance were each described in two of the 20 vignettes. Psychic Agitation was described in three vignettes. Dysphoric Mood and Marital/Relational Dysfunction were each described in four vignettes, and Family Dysfunction was described in five vignettes. The remaining 58 vignettes were each presented once, resulting in 80 impairment depictions across the 20 vignettes. These depictions did not include actual impairment terms, e.g., Dysphoric mood, or similar phrases, e.g., "dysphoria," except in five instances where it was pragmatically infeasible to avoid doing so. Specifically, the phrases "setting fire," "stealing," and "assault" were used in the Vignette 3, and the phrases "running away" and "lying" were used in Vignette 16. These exceptions did not inflate interrater reliability; however, the median true positive rate for the five impairments affected by these exceptions (93.8%) was equal to the rate for the entire set of 63 impairments (93.8%).

Appendix B: Empirical Research Articles

PATIENT IMPAIRMENT LEXICON

information not included in a vignette was assumed to be ruled out. Thus, for each patient, the data provided to raters approximated that which might be obtained via a structured interview. After reading each vignette, raters indicated which of the 63 impairments were present and then rated each selected one's severity.

To facilitate assessment of content validity, raters were also instructed to give feedback following the completion of the materials. Specifically, raters were asked to identify (a) any impairment definitions in the lexicon which seemed unclear or apparently overlapped with other impairments and (b) any additional potential impairment terms not included in the lexicon. Following the group administration session (3 hours), raters completed materials independently (in an average of 2.5 additional hours) and were paid after handing in their booklets. In the rare instances in which raters left an item blank, booklets were returned for completion.

Finally, six months later, five of the original raters were randomly selected to complete the materials a second time. Once again, for each identified patient, these five raters indicated which of the 63 impairments were present and then provided a severity rating for each one.

RESULTS

As previously stated, seven impairments were depicted more than once across the 20 vignettes. Results from these seven were summed and averaged to give them equivalent weight relative to the entire set of 63 impairments.

Interrater Reliability

Assessment began with evaluation of the entire 63 impairments as a set, using Cronbach alpha. Specifically, the 63 impairments were entered as "subjects" and the 16 raters as "items" in the data set. As such, Cronbach alpha provided an estimation of the extent to which all 63 impairments as a set were rated consistently by the 16 raters. When alpha was computed for presence or absence of impairments (scored as 1 or 0, respectively), $\alpha = .67$. When alpha was computed for the severity of impairments (scored as 0, 1, 2, 3, or 4), $\alpha = .86$.

Assessment of interrater reliability continued with analyses of true positives concerning the intended individual impairments across all 20 vignettes without regard to severity (0 = absent, 1 = present).[4] True positive percentages for the impairments ranged from 56.3%–100.0%, with a median of 93.8% (see Table 2). Next, true-negative percentages were calculated, based

---

[4]Three to five impairments were presented in each vignette, resulting in chance agreement rates regarding any one impairment ranging from 4.8% to 7.9%. Thus, the influence of chance on ratings was minimal, and true positives and negatives were used as reasonable estimates of interrater reliability.

on the fact that each impairment could potentially be selected with respect to each of the 20 vignettes. Thus, for the majority of impairments, a 100% true negative response would entail raters' abstaining from selection in 19 of the 20 vignettes (with selection in the remaining vignette constituting a true positive response). True negative percentages ranged from 86.1%–100.0%, with a median of 98.4% (see Table 2).

Interrater reliability of rated severity (i.e., 0 = absent, 4 = imminently dangerous) for each individual impairment was also examined (see Table 2). First, reliability was assessed as the extent to which raters' scores on the 4-point severity scale were identical to the intended severities depicted in the 20 vignettes. The percentages of agreement regarding these ratings of "correct" severity varied considerably across impairments (range = 6.3%–87.5%; $Mdn = 31.3\%$). Second, as a less conservative analysis, reliability was assessed as the extent to which ratings of severity were within one point above or below of the intended ratings of "correct" severity for each impairment in the 20 vignettes.[5] Agreement percentages regarding these "good" severity ratings were higher (range = 56.3%–100.0%; $Mdn = 87.6\%$).

Temporal Stability

Based on the over-all poor interrater reliability of rated severity for individual impairments at Time 1, the temporal stability of these ratings at Time 2 was not assessed. It was computed, however, regarding presence of the impairments versus their absence (true positives). Specifically, for each of the 63 impairments depicted, the five randomly selected raters' judgments at Times 1 and 2 were compared. For example, if all five raters made identical judgments regarding the presence versus absence of an impairment at Times 1 and 2, this resulted in 100% temporal stability; if only two of five raters made such identical judgments, this resulted in 40% temporal stability. Table 3 shows that, in general, temporal stability for the individual impairments was fair to good (range = 40%–100%; $Mdn = 100\%$).

Content Validity

Evaluation began with a qualitative assessment concerning the extent to which the Patient Impairment Lexicon's 63 impairments were relevant to and representative of all treatable mental health impairments. Raters offered no critical comments concerning exclusivity of impairment terms, and only four suggestions were made by only a few raters regarding additional potential terms in connection with the 20 case vignettes: (a) Psychological Treatment Noncompliance, (b) Deficient Memory Functioning, (c) Anger Man-

---

[5]This procedure involved one exception. Severity ratings of 0 were not considered "good" when the "correct" severity rating was 1 because ratings of 0 implied the absence of an impairment. Thus, ratings of 0 were not recoded.

TABLE 2
IMPAIRMENT ACCURACY ACROSS ALL 63 IMPAIRMENTS

Impairment[a]	Rated Severity (0–1)		Depicted Severity	Rated Severity (0–4)		
	% True Positive[b]	% True Negative[c]		M Obtained Severity	% Correct Severity[d]	% Good Severity[e]
Dissociative states[f]	100.0	100.0	2	2.94	25.0	81.3
Running away	100.0	100.0	3	2.50	37.5	87.5
Sexual trauma perpetrator	100.0	100.0	3	3.00	87.5	100.0
Uncontrolled gambling	100.0	100.0	2	2.75	31.3	93.8
Delusions (paranoid)	100.0	99.7	3	2.75	75.0	100.0
Somatization	100.0	99.7	1	1.94	31.3	75.0
School avoidance	100.0	99.3	1	2.37	6.3	56.3
Physical abuse perpetrator	100.0	99.0	3	3.00	62.5	100.0
Sexual performance deficit	100.0	99.0	2	1.94	25.0	93.8
Assaultiveness	100.0	98.4	4	3.62	68.8	93.8
Compulsions	100.0	98.4	3	2.25	25.0	75.0
Eating disorder	100.0	98.4	3	2.19	25.0	93.8
Medical treatment noncompliance	100.0	98.4	2	2.00	50.0	100.0
Manic thought/behavior	100.0	97.7	4	3.00	25.0	75.0
Phobia	100.0	97.4	2	2.81	12.5	93.8
Obsessions	100.0	97.0	3	2.37	12.5	75.0
Psychotic thought/behavior	100.0	95.7	4	3.12	18.1	93.8
Self-esteem deficit	100.0	94.7	2	2.06	56.3	100.0
Mood lability	100.0	93.1	2	2.12	25.0	100.0
Encopresis	93.8	100.0	1	1.19	75.0	93.8
Enuresis	93.8	100.0	1	1.37	62.5	87.5

(continued on next page)

[a]Impairments occur in only one vignette unless otherwise stated as averaged. [b]False negative percentages are simply the inverse of true positive percentages. Both are relative to the 63 intended impairments. [c]False positive percentages are simply the inverse of true negative percentages. Both are relative to the 20 potential citings of each impairment across the 20 vignettes. [d]Exact ratings were identical to depicted ratings. [e]Approximate ratings were within ± 1 point of depicted ratings. [f]Criteria for presentation order is first by descending order of true positive percentage, second by descending order of true negative percentages within true positive percentage order, and third alphabetically.

TABLE 2 (CONT'D)
IMPAIRMENT ACCURACY ACROSS ALL 63 IMPAIRMENTS

Impairment[a]	Rated Severity (0–1)		Rated Severity (0–4)			
	% True Positive[b]	% True Negative[c]	Depicted Severity	M Obtained Severity	% Correct Severity[d]	% Good Severity[e]
Gender dysphoria	93.8	100.0	2	1.69	31.3	87.6
Hallucinations	93.8	100.0	3	2.56	68.8	93.8
Physical abuse victim	93.8	100.0	2	2.31	25.0	87.6
Substance abuse	93.8	100.0	3	2.25	37.5	93.8
Suicidal thought/behavior	93.8	100.0	3	2.25	31.3	75.1
Promiscuity	93.8	99.7	2	2.81	18.8	81.3
Sexual trauma victim	93.8	99.7	2	2.12	56.3	93.9
Pathological grief	93.8	99.3	2	1.87	56.3	93.9
Self-mutilation	93.8	99.3	2	2.87	18.8	75.1
Emotional abuse perpetrator	93.8	98.7	2	2.19	25.0	93.8
Truancy	93.8	98.7	1	1.62	37.5	87.5
Concomitant medical condition	93.8	98.0	2	1.56	37.5	93.8
Uncontrolled buying	93.8	96.7	2	2.06	37.5	93.8
Oppositionalism	93.8	96.1	2	2.19	50.0	81.3
Emotional abuse victim	93.8	95.4	2	1.81	37.5	93.8
Alexithymia	93.8	95.1	2	1.87	31.3	81.3
Altered sleep (2 averaged)	93.8	93.4	1.5	1.47	25.0	100.0
Motor hyperactivity	93.8	93.4	2	2.25	50.0	87.6
Manipulative	93.8	92.8	1	1.31	62.5	93.8
Lying	93.8	92.4	1	1.81	25.0	87.5
Decreased concentration	93.8	91.1	2	1.81	62.5	93.8
Egocentricity (2 averaged)	93.8	87.9	2	1.75	12.5	100.0
Marital/relationship dysfunction (4 averaged)	92.2	93.0	2	1.72	12.5	87.6
Inadequate healthcare skills	87.5	97.0	1	1.50	31.3	93.8

(continued on next page)

TABLE 2 (Cont'd)

IMPAIRMENT ACCURACY ACROSS ALL 63 IMPAIRMENTS

Impairment[a]	Rated Severity (0–1)		Depicted Severity	Rated Severity (0–4)		
	% True Positive[b]	% True Negative[c]		M Obtained Severity	% Correct Severity[d]	% Good Severity[e]
Delusions (nonparanoid)	87.5	95.7	4	2.75	18.8	81.3
Social withdrawal	87.5	91.5	1	2.00	12.5	68.8
Externalization and blame	87.5	88.2	2	1.50	25.0	87.6
Family dysfunction (5 averaged)	83.8	97.9	1.8	1.76	12.5	100.0
Dysphoric mood (4 averaged)	82.8	91.4	2	1.44	18.8	93.9
Stealing	81.3	100.0	2	2.12	31.3	68.9
Tantrums	81.3	99.3	2	1.56	37.5	81.3
Inadequate self-maintenance skills (2 averaged)	78.1	88.9	2	1.91	25.0	93.8
Psychic agitation (3 averaged)	77.1	86.1	1.3	1.58	12.5	68.8
Psychomotor retardation	75.0	99.7	2	1.31	56.3	75.1
Educational performance deficit	75.0	95.4	2	1.37	43.8	75.1
Homicidal thought/behavior	68.8	100.0	4	2.44	37.5	68.8
Pathological guilt	68.8	99.3	1	1.44	18.8	81.3
Fire setting	62.5	100.0	4	2.44	56.3	62.6
Learning disability	62.5	99.3	1	1.00	31.3	93.8
Medical risk factor	62.5	98.4	2	1.56	18.8	56.3
Uncommunicativeness	62.5	91.8	1	.69	56.3	100.0
Sexual object choice dysfunction	56.3	97.7	2	1.62	6.3	56.3

[a] Impairments occur in only one vignette unless otherwise stated as averaged. [b] False negative percentages are simply the inverse of true positive percentages. Both are relative to the 63 intended impairments. [c] False positive percentages are simply the inverse of true negative percentages. Both are relative to the 20 potential citings of each impairment across the 20 vignettes. [d] Exact ratings were identical to depicted ratings. [e] Approximate ratings were within ±1 point of depicted ratings. [f] Criteria for presentation order is first by descending order of true positive percentage, second by descending order of true negative percentages within true positive percentage order, and third alphabetically.

560   L. L. KLEWICKI, *ET AL.*

agement Problem, and (d) Neuropsychological Dysfunction. Thus, raters generally judged the impairments to describe comprehensively all treatable mental health impairments, at least with reference to these 20 depicted patients.

Content validity is also reflected by the extent to which a measure's items exhibit accuracy, specificity, and clarity (Haynes, *et al.*, 1995). To this end, assessment of content validity continued with an examination of im-

TABLE 3
TEST-RETEST IMPAIRMENT ACCURACY ACROSS ALL 63 IMPAIRMENTS

Impairment[a]	% Agreement[b]	Impairment	% Agreement
Alexithymia[c]	100.0	Suicidal thought/behavior	100.0
Assaultiveness	100.0	Uncontrolled gambling	100.0
Compulsions	100.0	Altered sleep[d]	90.0
Concomitant medical condition	100.0	Delusions (nonparanoid)	80.0
Decreased concentration	100.0	Dysphoric mood[d]	80.0
Delusions (paranoid)	100.0	Egocentricity[d]	80.0
Dissociative states	100.0	Emotional abuse victim	80.0
Eating disorder	100.0	Externalization and blame	80.0
Emotional abuse perpetrator	100.0	Hallucinations	80.0
Encopresis	100.0	Manipulativeness	80.0
Enuresis	100.0	Medical risk factor	80.0
Gender dysphoria	100.0	Obsessions	80.0
Inadequate healthcare skills	100.0	Psychomotor retardation	80.0
Lying	100.0	Psychotic thought/behavior	80.0
Manic thought/behavior	100.0	Self-esteem deficit	80.0
Medical treatment noncompliance	100.0	Sexual object choice dysfunction	80.0
Mood lability	100.0	Sexual performance deficit	80.0
Motor hyperactivity	100.0	Stealing	80.0
Oppositionalism	100.0	Truancy	80.0
Pathological grief	100.0	Uncontrolled buying	80.0
Phobia	100.0	Educational performance deficit	76.0
Physical abuse perpetrator	100.0	Fire setting	76.0
Physical abuse victim	100.0	Homicidal thought/behavior	76.0
Promiscuity	100.0	Pathological guilt	76.0
Running away	100.0	Tantrums	76.0
School avoidance	100.0	Family dysfunction[d]	72.0
Self-mutilation	100.0	Inadequate self-maintenance skills[d]	70.0
Sexual trauma perpetrator	100.0	Marital/relationship dysfunction[d]	70.0
Sexual trauma victim	100.0	Psychic agitation[d]	67.0
Social withdrawal	100.0	Learning dysfunction	40.0
Somatization	100.0	Uncommunicativeness	40.0
Substance abuse	100.0		

[a]Impairments occur in only one vignette unless otherwise stated as averaged. [b]Percent agreement was calculated using a 0–1 scale, i.e., either the rater depicted the impairment as occurring or not occurring. [c]Criteria for presentation order is first by descending order of percentage agreement and second alphabetically. [d]This impairment occurred more than once in the 20 vignettes. Ratings were summed and averaged to give equivalent weight relative to the entire set of 63 impairments.

Appendix B: Empirical Research Articles **227**

PATIENT IMPAIRMENT LEXICON 561

TABLE 4
PROPOSED EXPLANATIONS FOR RATERS' 10 CONSISTENT FALSE POSITIVE RATINGS OF IMPAIRMENT

False Positive	Vignette	%[a]	Proposed Explanation of Error[b]
Vignette Problem[c]			
Altered sleep †	6	87.5	The identified patient (age 32) does state "he . . . 'only got about three hours of sleep' per night over the entire week. . ."
Egocentricity	3	87.5	The identified patient (age 41) does show empathic failure regarding his setting fire to his girlfriend's trailer by stating, "If she was too dumb to wake up when she smelled smoke, it would have served her right."
Emotional abuse victim	9	81.3	The identified patient (age 7) does acknowledge emotional abuse by stating that "John (baby sitter) says I'm too dumb to do things myself. He must help me or I can't do things."
Decreased concentration	15	62.5	The identified patient (age 14) does state she is "too tired to keep my mind on school work—especially after lunch."
Impairment Term[c]			
Lying	13	62.5	The identified patient (age 40) "denies engaging in sexual intercourse" with his daughter. Telling one lie currently meets the definitional criteria. Thus, the definition should be changed to refer to a pervasive pattern of lying (versus only an occasional lie).
Psychotic thought/behavior	2	75.0	The identified patient (age 24) does state "demons from the movie I watched last week . . . want to get me. . ." This delusion is peculiar ideation, which meets the definitional criteria. Thus, the term's definition should be changed to distinguish peculiar ideations from delusions.

(continued on next page)

[a] Refers to the percent of raters who erroneously depicted the specified impairment as existing in the given vignette. [b] Proposed explanation of errors is based upon discussion with the raters. Quotes are taken from the vignettes. [c] Refers to the proposed reason for the error. † Definitions are as follows: Altered sleep = Any disruption of the normal 24-hour sleep-wake cycle, including insomnia, hypersomnia, early morning awakening, or night terrors; Egocentricity = Excessive evaluation of things in terms of one's self and one's personal interests (for example, excessive self-importance, arrogance, and empathic failures with others; Emotional abuse victim = The victim of deliberate nonphysical acts, including verbal abuse and emotional neglect, that are psychologically damaging; Decreased concentration = Any observed or reported reduction in ability to direct one's thoughts or efforts to sustain attention; Lying = Deliberate falsification; Psychotic thought/behavior = Incoherence, repeated derailment or loosening of associations, marked illogicality, peculiar ideation, or marked poverty of thought; and/or grossly disorganized behaviors that may be dangerous or unexplainable.

TABLE 4 (CONT'D)

PROPOSED EXPLANATIONS FOR RATERS' 10 CONSISTENT FALSE POSITIVE RATINGS OF IMPAIRMENT

Raters' Error[c]	Vignette	%[a]	Proposed Explanation of Error[b]
False Positive			
Decreased concentration †	11	62.5	The identified patient (age 9) "has always been really distractible" and "frequently fails to complete assigned tasks." Raters failed to note that she has not experienced any reduction in concentration (but rather has always functioned at this level).
Dysphoric mood	8	62.5	The identified patient "speaks somewhat slowly," "delays at times before responding," and has had "recent trouble concentrating." Raters failed to note that she "feel[s] fine." They apparently are assuming a diagnosis of Depression, but no Dysphoric Mood is present.
Externalization and blame	3	62.5	The identified patient states "nobody kicks me out and gets away with it, so I figured I'd teach her a lesson. ..." Raters failed to note that he was not blaming anyone for his actions but simply acknowledged being angered by another.
Marital/relationship dysfunction	3	62.5	The identified patient states "I'm glad it's over between us." Raters failed to note that there is no current relationship to treat and no desire for reconciliation.

[a] Refers to the percent of raters who erroneously depicted the specified impairment as existing in the given vignette. [b] Proposed explanation of errors is based upon discussion with the raters. Quotes are taken from the vignettes. [c] Refers to the proposed reason for the error. † Definitions are as follows: Decreased concentration = Any observed or reported reduction in ability to direct one's thoughts or efforts to sustain attention; Dysphoric mood = Conscious and apparent psychic suffering characterized by sadness, gloominess, despair, or despondency; Externalization and blame = Constant or inappropriate attributing of an intrapsychic function to an interpersonal experience (for example, "I did what I did because 'he,' 'she,' or 'they' ..."); Marital or relationship dysfunction = Impaired marital or relationship functioning (due to either or both partners).

PATIENT IMPAIRMENT LEXICON   563

pairments that were consistently not identified although intentionally depicted (false negative) and those which were identified but not intentionally
depicted (false positive). The only consistent false negative was Sexual Object Choice Dysfunction, i.e., all other intended impairments were rated by
10 or more of the 16 raters, see Table 2. No impairments were consistently
cited as false positives across all 20 vignettes (see Table 2). There were ten
instances, however, in which 10 or more of the 16 raters cited the same false
positive impairment within a given vignette. Examination of these ten false
positives suggested three potential causes: (a) a given vignette actually depicted an impairment not intended by the authors, (b) definition of a given
impairment term was ambiguous, or (c) the raters made an error. Table 4
lists the 10 impairments with the corresponding proposed explanation for
each of these false positives.

DISCUSSION

Evaluation of treatment efficacy requires the use of a reliable and valid
common nomenclature describing the full range of treatable mental health
impairments. The current study's results provide preliminary support for the
use of the Patient Impairment Lexicon as such a nomenclature. We found
that student clinicians showed moderate to strong agreement in their use of
the lexicon, with moderate to high true positive percentages and high true
negative percentages across all 63 impairments. These findings suggest that
the majority of raters not only consistently identified any given impairment
when it was present but also consistently discriminated among impairment
terms. This is particularly significant given that raters had no previous exposure to the lexicon and only minimal training (one example) prior to completing their ratings.

Whereas interrater reliability regarding the presence versus absence of
individual impairments was moderate to excellent, it was generally poor for
rated severity of impairment (i.e., 1 = distressing, 4 = imminently dangerous).
This might have been partially due to the fact that raters' training was minimal. Specifically, the wide variance in percentage of agreement with intended severities (range = 6.3%—87.5%) suggested that raters might not have
been using these ratings of severity as instructed. Specifically, ratings of severity are designed to reflect extent to which a given impairment compromises the patient's normal functioning. Feedback from raters, however, suggested that some might have used severities to rate how upsetting an impairment was to the patient and/or how many behaviors were linked with a giv-
en impairment. Thus, for example, a rater might have assigned a severity of
4, i.e., imminently dangerous, to the impairment Altered Sleep if the patient
was not sleeping at all and extremely upset about it. This would be incorrect, however, because Altered Sleep can never be imminently dangerous,

i.e., life threatening. Clearly, researchers must ensure that instructions regarding severity of impairment are clarified, to optimize content validity and provide a more accurate evaluation of these ratings.

Interrater agreement regarding the entire 63 impairments as a set was moderate to high ($\alpha = .67$—$.86$). The higher internal consistency associated with the more quantitative 0- to 4-point scale suggests that using quantitative ratings of severity improved reliability as compared to simply using categories (0- to 1-point scale). The poor interrater agreement regarding individual ratings of severity of impairment discussed above, however, limits the generalizability of these findings regarding the entire set of impairments. It is possible, for example, that the high internal consistency ($\alpha = .86$) was due to all raters using the 4-point severity ratings in similar fashion although incorrectly. Regardless, in light of the need for exceptional reliability ($\alpha > .90$; Nunnally & Bernstein, 1994) when assessing individual (versus group) differences, further refinement of the lexicon is clearly needed. Still, regarding judgments of the presence versus absence of an impairment, 70% of the impairment terms had true positive rates of 90% or higher, and 94% of impairment terms had comparable true negative rates. Together, these findings support the potential of the lexicon as a useful tool for clinical assessment.

Preliminary assessment of temporal stability provided additional support for the use of the Patient Impairment Lexicon as a reliable diagnostic nomenclature. Raters showed at least 80% agreement regarding 85% of impairment terms, and the lengthy intertest interval (six months) reduced the possibility that these findings were confounded by memory effects. Research is needed, however, to assess the temporal stability of rated severity.

We also assessed the lexicon's content validity. Whereas content validity has many facets (Haynes, et al., 1995), our study addressed a few central ones. For example, our results suggested that the lexicon's 63 impairments were representative of and relevant to the domain of treatable mental health impairments (Nunnally & Bernstein, 1994). Specifically, when assessing 20 cases depicting patients evidencing 18 widely divergent diagnoses, only four suggestions were made (by only a few raters) for additional potential impairment terms not covered in the lexicon. Furthermore, closer inspection of these four indicated that each was already addressed by an existing impairment term. Psychological Treatment Noncompliance was suggested but is redundant, given that Medical Treatment Noncompliance is meant to cover any behavioral or physical health issue. Deficient Memory Functioning was proposed but can readily be subsumed under Decreased Concentration, which covers "any observed or reported reduction in ability to direct one's thoughts..." (Goodman, et al., 1996, p. 172). The third proposed additional impairment, Anger Management Problem, is already represented at a more specific level (e.g., Assaultiveness, Tantrums). Finally, Neuropsycholog-

PATIENT IMPAIRMENT LEXICON   565

ical Dysfunction was suggested but is readily subsumed under Concomitant Medical Condition, particularly if one recalls that the lexicon's terms describe mental health impairments that are treatable. Thus, these four suggestions seemed to reflect the minimal exposure and training raters had rather than an actual need for additional terms. Together, these qualitative findings suggest that the lexicon's 63 original terms adequately represent the domain of treatable mental health impairment. They also suggest that training must be more extensive than the minimal instructions provided raters in the current study. Given the extensive study typically associated with mastering diagnostic systems (e.g., Spitzer, Gibbon, Skodol, Williams, & First, 1994), however, these initial results with the lexicon are promising.

Content validity was also evaluated via inspection of false negatives and false positives. Only one consistent false negative was identified (Sexual Object Choice Dysfunction). This impairment was depicted in Vignette 13 (see Table 1), which also involved the impairment Sexual Trauma Perpetrator. Thus, many raters apparently erroneously presumed that inappropriate sexual object choice is inferred by Sexual Trauma Perpetrator. These two impairments, however, can occur together or independently. In Vignette 13, for example, the sexual trauma was directed at a child, representing a concomitantly inappropriate choice of sexual object. Further development and research will need to eliminate this ambiguity by highlighting the mutual exclusivity of these two impairments.

There were also ten instances in which the majority of raters identified the same false positive impairment, i.e., one not intended by the authors, in a given vignette. When interpreting these findings, it should first be noted that each rater could have potentially give close to 1200 false positive responses across the 20 vignettes. Second, only four of the "false" positive responses were legitimate errors (see Table 4). Four others represented correct identification of unintended depictions of impairment due to faulty vignette construction by the authors. Thus, including these four responses in the false positive calculations actually resulted in slightly underestimating raters' accuracy. The remaining two "false" positives actually reflected ambiguities in definitions of impairment terms and these ambiguities will be eliminated in development of and research of the Patient Impairment Lexicon. Given that this was the raters' first exposure to the lexicon and that roughly 1200 false positive responses were possible, the four actual false positive errors represent relatively minor limitations to the accuracy and utility of this system. Therefore, false positive assessment generally lends additional support to the content validity of the lexicon.

The current findings must be interpreted in light of several methodological limitations. Whereas the use of vignettes permitted a more standardized basis for assessment of interrater reliability, this limits the extent to which these findings are generalizable to actual events and real individuals. For example, actual patient assessment would require a standardized method of data collection (e.g., a structured interview). Thus, the current study is only a first step (Hjortso, *et al.*, 1989) in evaluating the lexicon. Another limitation of the present study is that all diagnostic categories as presented in the DSM-III–R were not represented in the 20 given vignettes. Thus, even though the 20 vignettes depicted a wide array of diagnoses, it is not known how well the current findings may generalize to types of patients not presented in the vignettes. Furthermore, the Patient Impairment Lexicon should also be evaluated with reference to the DSM-IV, which includes some significant changes from its predecessor. The current findings are also statistically limited by the range of psychometric evaluation involved, i.e., interrater reliability, temporal stability, and content validity. At the very least, construct and criterion-related validity (Nunnally & Bernstein, 1994) must also be examined. Such research is currently underway, specifically comparing the lexicon with the DSM-IV. In addition, those facets of psychometric evaluation examined in the current study, e.g., content validity, require more comprehensive scrutiny (Haynes, *et al.*, 1995).

Some might also cite the use of graduate students as raters (whose performance might not generalize to that of professionals) as another potential methodological limitation. Several studies suggest that professionals have more experience with actual patients and thus might assess them more accurately (Greve, 1993; Sharf & Lucas, 1993) and reliably (Maurer, Alexander, Callahan, Bailey, & Dambrot, 1991). If so, the current findings might actually underestimate reliability when the lexicon is used by professionals. Other research suggests, however, that there is no difference in rated accuracy between professionals and graduate students (Omer, Dar, Wainberg, & Grossbard, 1994), especially when both groups receive the same training with regard to an assessment measure (Axelrod, Greve, & Goldman, 1994). In either case, using graduate students does not appear to be a major methodological limitation.

Despite its limitations, the current study provides preliminary support for the Patient Impairment Lexicon as a useful clinical tool for communicating treatment needs within managed care systems. Specifically, it appears to be a useful nomenclature consisting of comprehensive, mutually exclusive, and discrete impairment terms with quantitative ratings of severity. Moreover, the system appears to be readily grasped and applied even after only minimal training. As such, it has potential for augmenting the DSM-IV's diagnostic system and aiding in effective treatment planning and research of outcomes. With today's growing emphasis on managed care, the need for clinical tools such as the lexicon can only be expected to increase.

PATIENT IMPAIRMENT LEXICON

REFERENCES

AMERICAN PSYCHIATRIC ASSOCIATION. (1952) *Diagnostic and statistical manual of mental disorders*. Washington, DC: Author.

AMERICAN PSYCHIATRIC ASSOCIATION. (1987) *Diagnostic and statistical manual of mental disorders*. (3rd ed., Rev.) Washington, DC: Author.

AMERICAN PSYCHIATRIC ASSOCIATION. (1994) *Diagnostic and statistical manual of mental disorders*. (4th ed.) Washington, DC: Author.

ANDERSEN, S. M., & HARTHORN, B. H. (1989) The diagnostic knowledge inventory: a measure of knowledge about psychiatric diagnosis. *Journal of Clinical Psychology*, 45, 999-1013.

ATROM, J., THORELL, L. H., HOMLUND, U., & D'ELIA, G. (1993) Handshaking, personality, and psychopathology in psychiatric patients: a reliability and correlational study. *Perceptual and Motor Skills*, 77, 1171-1186.

AXELROD, B. N., GREVE, K. W., & GOLDMAN, R. S. (1994) Comparison of four Wisconsin Card Sorting Test scoring guides with novice raters. *Assessment*, 1, 115-121.

BARLOW, D. H. (1994) Psychological interventions in the era of managed competition. *Clinical Psychology: Science and Practice*, 1, 109-122.

CALHOUN, K. S., MORAS, K., PILKONIS, P., & REHM, L. P. (1998) Empirically supported treatments: implications for training. *Journal of Consulting and Clinical Psychology*, 66, 151-162.

CHRISMAN, A. K., LANCASTER, M., ROSS, R., AINSWORTH, T. L., HEMMINGS, K., SHAFFER, I. A. (1996) Towards a standard documentation for behavioral health. *Journal of Practical Psychiatry and Behavioral Health*, 2, 105-110.

CLARK, L. A., WATSON, D., & REYNOLDS, S. (1995) Diagnosis and classification of psychopathology: challenges to the current system and future directions. *Annual Review of Psychology*, 46, 121-153.

COLEMAN, M. J., CARPENER, J. T., WATERNAUX, C., LEVY, D. L., SHENTON, M. E., PERRY, J., MEDOFF, D., WONG, H., MONOACH, D., MEYER, P., O'BRIAN, C., VALENTINO, C., ROBINSON, D., SMITH, M., MAKOWSKI, D., & HOLZMAN, P. S. (1993) The Thought Disorder Index: a reliability study. *Psychological Assessment*, 5, 336-342.

EVENSON, R. C., & BOYD, M. A. (1993) The St. Louis Inventory of Community Living Skills. *Psychosocial Rehabilitation Journal*, 17, 93-99.

GOLDFRIED, M. R., & WOLFE, B. E. (1998) Toward a more clinically valid approach to therapy research. *Journal of Consulting and Clinical Psychology*, 66, 143-150.

GOODMAN, M., BROWN, J., & DEITZ, P. (1992) *Managing managed care: a mental health practitioner's survival guide*. Washington, DC: American Psychiatric Press.

GOODMAN, M., BROWN, J., & DEITZ, P. (1996) *Managing managed care: a handbook for mental health professionals*. (2nd ed.) Washington, DC: American Psychiatric Press.

GREVE, K. W. (1993) Can perspective responses on the Wisconsin Card Sorting Test be scored accurately? *Archives of Clinical Neuropsychology*, 8, 511-517.

HASIN, D., & LINK, B. (1988) Age and recognition of depression: implications for a cohort effect in major depression. *Psychological Medicine*, 18, 683-688.

HAYES, S. C., WILSON, K. G., GIFFORD, E. V., FOLLETTE, V. M., & STROSAHL, K. (1996) Experiential avoidance and behavioral disorders: a functional dimensional approach to diagnosis and treatment. *Journal of Consulting and Clinical Psychology*, 64, 1152-1168.

HAYNES, S. N., RICHARD, D. C. S., & KUBANY, E. S. (1995) Content validity in psychological assessment: a functional approach to concepts and methods. *Psychological Assessment*, 7, 238-247.

HEUMANN, K. A., & MOREY, L. C. (1990) Reliability of categorical and dimensional judgments of personality disorder. *American Journal of Psychiatry*, 147, 498-500.

HEVERLY, M. A., FITT, D. X., & NEWMAN, F. L. (1984) Constructing case vignettes for evaluating clinical judgment: an empirical model. *Evaluation and Program Planning*, 7, 45-55.

HJORTSO, S., BUTLER, B., CLEMMENSEN, L., JEPSEN, P. W., KASTRUP, M., VILMAR, T., & BECH, P. (1989) The use of case vignettes in studies of interrater reliability of psychiatric target syndromes and diagnoses: a comparison of ICD–8, ICD–10 and DSM–III. *Acta Psychiatrica Scandinavica*, 80, 632-638.

KAPLAN, C. (1993) Reliability and validity of test-session behavior observations: putting the horse before the cart. *Journal of Psychoeducational Assessment*, 11, 314-322.

LANZA, M. L., & CARIFIO, J. (1992) Use of a panel of experts to establish validity for patient assault vignettes. *Evaluation Review*, 16, 82-92.

LILIENFELD, S. O., WALDMAN, I. D., & ISRAEL, A. C. (1994) A critical examination of the use of the term and concept of "comorbidity" in psychopathology research. *Clinical Psychology: Science and Practice*, 1, 71-83.

MARWIT, S. J. (1996) Reliability of diagnosing complicated grief: a preliminary investigation. *Journal of Consulting and Clinical Psychology*, 64, 563-568.

MAURER, T. J., ALEXANDER, R. A., CALLAHAN, C. M., BAILEY, J. J., & DAMBROT, F. H. (1991) Methodological and psychometric issues in setting cutoff scores using the Angoff method. *Personnel Psychology*, 44, 235-262.

NORCROSS, J. C., KARG, R. S., & PROCHASKA, J. O. (1997) Clinical psychologists and managed care: some data from the Division 12 membership. *The Clinical Psychologist*, 50, 4-8.

NUNNALLY, J. C., & BERNSTEIN, I. (1994) *Psychometric theory*. San Francisco, CA: McGraw-Hill.

OMER, H., DAR, R., WAINBERG, B., & GROSSBARD, O. (1994) A process scale for impact-promoting activities. *Psychotherapy Research*, 4, 34-42.

PONSFORD, J., & KINSELLA, G. (1991) The use of a rating scale of attentional behavior. *Neuropsychological Rehabilitation*, 1, 241-257.

SECHREST, L., McKNIGHT, P., & McKNIGHT, K. (1996) Calibration of measures for psychotherapy outcome studies. *American Psychologist*, 51, 1065-1071.

SHARF, R. S., & LUCAS, M. (1993) An assessment of a computerized simulation of counseling skills. *Counselor Education and Supervision*, 43, 254-266.

SHEPHERD, M., BROOKE, E. M., COOPER, J. E., & LIN, T. (1968) An experimental approach of psychiatric diagnosis. *Acta Psychiatrica Scandinavica*, 44(Suppl. 201), 7-89.

SORENSEN, J. L., HARGREAVES, W. A., & FRIEDLANDER, S. (1982) Child global rating scales: selecting a measure of client functioning in a large mental health system. *Evaluation and Program Planning*, 5, 337-347.

SPITZER, R. L., GIBBON, M., SKODOL, A. E., WILLIAMS, J. B. W., & FIRST, M. B. (1994) *DSM–IV casebook: a learning companion to the diagnostic and statistical manual of mental disorders.* (4th ed.) Washington, DC: American Psychiatric Press.

TAUBE, C. A., LEE, E. S., & FORTHOFER, R. N. (1984) Diagnosis related groups for mental disorders, alcoholism and drug abuse: evaluation and alternatives. *Hospital and Community Psychiatry*, 35, 452-455.

WIDIGER, T. A., & FORD-BLACK, M. M. (1994) Diagnoses and disorders. *Clinical Psychology: Science and Practice*, 1, 84-87.

WULFURT, E., GREENWAY, D. E., & DOUGHER, M. J. (1996) A logical functional analysis of reinforcement-based disorders: alcoholism and pedophilia. *Journal of Consulting and Clinical Psychology*, 64, 1140-1151.

Accepted July 27, 1998.

APPENDIX
Case Presentation 7: "Nancy"

Reason For Referral

Nancy, a 47 year old African-American female, has come to see you because "I just can't stop washing my hands." She is single, has never been married, and lives alone in a nearby apartment complex. You interview Nancy and obtain the following information:

History

Nancy is a computer technician who enjoys her work and has received favorable evaluations throughout the eight years at her current position. While she considers several fellow employees to be her "good friends," and she does attend the occasional work-related social functions, "I've always been somewhat of an introvert." Nancy reports that for the past few months, she has been washing her hands "probably 25 or 30 times a day." She tells you that she is repeatedly troubled by the thought that "I might get AIDS by touching something contaminated." The only way that she can obtain relief and/or stop the intrusive thoughts is to wash her hands repeatedly. These problems began for Nancy four months ago when another employee left work on disability "and it turned out he has AIDS." Nancy gradually became preoccupied with her AIDS fears and after some time "found that washing my hands seemed to help." This began slowly but increased as the repetitive thoughts became more frequent. "For all I know, half the office has AIDS. I know it's not likely, but anything is *possible*, and that's what makes me nuts!" Nancy states further, "No matter how hard I try, I just can't get beyond this. I feel like I don't have any control over it."

When you ask for more information regarding her dread of contracting AIDS, she explains that these thoughts and accompanying anxiety start "first thing in the morning." They quickly gain intensity unless she washes and dries her hands "five or six times in a row." This puts her at ease for a while, but the thoughts often return "within an hour or two;" her anxiety then increases again until she washes. The urge to wash is not as strong at home, but "the only time I'm totally ok is when I go to sleep at night with the gloves on." (Because her hands have become so dry and chapped, she is using large amounts of hand cream and wearing gloves to bed.) Nancy states she is aware that "you supposedly can't get it from just touching things, but washing my hands helps me cope. Still, I know it's crazy, and it's starting to help less and less." Apparently no one knows yet at work, "but someone is bound to find out, or at least ask why my hands are so chapped. I just have to get help!"

Clinical Presentation

Nancy presents as a casually dressed, neatly groomed female of average height and weight. She sits forward in her chair throughout the interview, wringing her hands frequently, and she appears to be shivering slightly. When asked if she is cold, she says "I guess maybe a little, but I think it's more my nerves." She is alert, oriented, and her speech is coherent, but her tone suggests a tense worried mood. Nancy exhibits above average intelligence. Her hands are badly chapped and her fingernails are clipped extremely short. She is very cooperative, and she answers each of your questions in minute detail being careful to include facts such as times and dates.

Assessment Assumptions

The psychiatric symptoms are not organic, and there is no substance abuse.

Instructions

Please complete all the questions that follow with respect to this case regarding *NANCY ONLY*. Remember that information not mentioned should be assumed to be nonapplicable to this case. Assume that all symptoms and/or relevant information are reported in the case description.

Appendix B: Empirical Research Articles

Patient Impairment Lexicon: A Validation Study

Christopher A. Leucht, Jeffrey P. Bjorck,
and Lisa L. Klewicki
Fuller Theological Seminary

Michael Goodman
UCLA School of Medicine

Growth of managed behavioral health organizations (MBHOs) has increased the need for a standardized diagnostic language. The Patient Impairment Lexicon (PIL; Goodman, Brown, & Deitz, 1992, 1996) is intended to address this need. Augmenting previous psychometric assessment (Klewicki, Bjorck, Leucht, & Goodman, 1998), the current study evaluated the PIL's construct validity. Sixteen raters completed impairment inventories; diagnoses based on the *Diagnostic and Statistical Manual of Mental Disorders*, Third Edition, Revised (DSM-III-R; American Psychiatric Association, 1987); and independent measures of psychiatric functioning for patients in 20 vignettes. Overall rater accuracy was significantly higher for PIL impairments than for diagnoses. As predicted, there were positive correlations between PIL impairments and psychiatric functioning for all 20 vignettes, 11 of which were significant. Results remained significant after controlling variance due to: (a) raters' past experience with similar patients and (b) vignette imaginability. Findings are discussed in terms of MBHO applications and future PIL research. © 1999 John Wiley & Sons, Inc. J Clin Psychol 55: 1567–1582, 1999.

With the rise in number and influence of managed behavioral health organizations (MBHOs), utilization reviewers are exerting increasing control over decisions regarding length and extent of mental health treatment (Goodman, Brown, & Deitz, 1992). Thus, clinicians must now be able not only to formulate appropriate treatment plans but also to

---

This article is based on a dissertation completed by Christopher A. Leucht under the direction of Jeffrey P. Bjorck at the Graduate School of Psychology, Fuller Theological Seminary. Thanks go to Richard L. Gorsuch for providing feedback on an earlier version of this article. We also acknowledge the helpful comments of Susan Noel and two anonymous reviewers.

Correspondence concerning this article should be addressed to Jeffrey P. Bjorck, Ph.D., Graduate School of Psychology, Fuller Theological Seminary, 180 North Oakland Avenue, Pasadena, CA 91101.

Reproduced with permission of the authors and publisher from:
Leucht C. A., Bjorck J. P., Klewicki L. L.: Patient Impairment Lexicon: A Validation Study. *Journal of Clinical Psychology* 55:1567–1582, 1999. Copyright © 1999 John Wiley & Sons, Inc.

effectively communicate the necessity of such treatment to reviewers. Given these circumstances, a universal, comprehensive diagnostic nomenclature is clearly needed to facilitate communication regarding patients' needs.[1] Such a standardized common language could also provide a logical basis for treatment plan development and generate reliable data for ongoing research regarding the quality of care (Chrisman, Lancaster, Ross, Ainsworth, Hemmings, & Shaffer1996). To accomplish these goals, however, this nomenclature would need to provide at least the following: (a) comprehensive coverage of all types of mental health problems; (b) intelligibility for all types of mental health professionals and utilization reviewers, independent of training level; and (c) applicability to all situations where mental health care is provided.

An obvious choice for a diagnostic nomenclature to meet these needs is the *Diagnostic and Statistical Manual of Medical Disorders*, Fourth Edition (DSM-IV; American Psychiatric Association, 1994). Not only does the DSM-IV provide the official diagnostic language for both psychiatrists and psychologists, but it is also frequently used by social workers, marriage and family counselors, and medical personnel. The authors of DSM-IV acknowledge, however, that this system has some clear limitations. For example, mental disorder categories are not assumed to be completely discrete, either from each other or from no disorder (p. xxii). Clark, Watson, and Reynolds (1995) note particularly strong overlap among diagnostic criteria for avoidant personality disorder and social phobia, antisocial personality disorder and substance abuse, mood disorders and borderline personality disorder, and schizotypal disorder and schizophrenia.

A second DSM-IV limitation concerns the fact that "individuals sharing a diagnosis are likely to be heterogeneous even in regard to defining features of the diagnosis" (p. xxii). Several recent authors (e. g., Clark et al., 1995; Follette & Houts, 1996; Hayes, Wilson, Gifford, Follette, & Strosahl, 1996; Wulfert, Greenway & Dougher, 1996) have critiqued the heterogeneity within DSM-IV categories. They often begin by citing the DSM-IV Task Force's admission that "there are more than 100 different ways for the criteria of Borderline Personality Disorder to be met" (Frances, First, & Pincus, 1995, p. 19). Clark et al. summarize results from several clinical studies finding great heterogeneity in patients with diagnoses from many diagnostic groupings (i.e., psychotic disorders, eating disorders, substance-related disorders, personality disorders, anxiety disorders, and mood disorders).

Follette and Houts (1996) have noted that whereas each successive edition of DSM has included more diagnostic categories, this growth has not apparently been accompanied by a corresponding growth in insight into the nature of mental disorders. Similarly, Clark et al. (1995) raise the concern that despite the large number of DSM-IV diagnoses, a sizable proportion of mental health patients still do not meet criteria in any existing category and are assigned a "not otherwise specified" (NOS) diagnosis. In support of this assertion, Clark and colleagues cite examples of clinical studies of depressive disorders, dissociative disorders, and personality disorders in which NOS diagnoses have been more prevalent than any standard diagnosis.

The overlap among many categories and great heterogeneity within them, the growing number of diagnostic categories, and the prevalence of NOS diagnoses are all indeed problematic aspects of the DSM-IV nomenclature. In addition, this terminology does little to facilitate communication regarding MBHOs' central concern, "Why is treatment

---

[1] In the present study, the word *patient* is used as a general reference to someone who uses mental health services, regardless of setting. Thus, in the present study a patient could be a participant in various forms of treatment, including inpatient or outpatient psychiatric care, outpatient psychotherapy, community-based mental health interventions, or drug/alcohol rehabilitation.

Appendix B: Empirical Research Articles

needed?" For example, whereas ten patients in a psychiatric unit might all be diagnosed with "major depression," each one might present with particular problems requiring unique treatment plans (Goodman, Brown, & Deitz, 1996). To their credit, the authors of DSM-IV acknowledge that a "diagnosis is only the first step in a comprehensive evaluation. To formulate an adequate treatment plan, the clinician will invariably require considerable information . . . beyond that required to make a DSM-IV diagnosis" (p. xxv). This need for additional information, combined with the limitations described above, have led many MBHOs to generate their own idiosyncratic systems for classifying and determining mental health treatment needs (Newman, 1996). Not only has this proliferation of systems increased confusion regarding treatment issues, but it has also hindered wide-scale treatment outcomes research. Clearly, a "single standard measure" (Sechrest, McKnight, & McKnight, 1996, p. 1070) for classifying patient impairments could facilitate communication as well as research efforts (Calhoun, Moras, Pilkonis, & Rehm, 1998; Goldfried & Wolfe, 1998).

The Patient Impairment Lexicon

The Patient Impairment Lexicon (PIL) was developed by Goodman et al. (1992) to provide a comprehensive diagnostic nomenclature, expressly designed to facilitate standardized communication and research. The original PIL was comprised of 65 operationally defined mental health impairment terms that were intended to comprehensively list all potential mental health treatment foci. Specifically, this nomenclature was designed to directly address the question "Why is treatment needed?" Revision of the PIL resulted in a current lexicon containing 63 terms (Haynes, Richard, & Kubany, 1995). The lexicon, consisting of the 63 terms and their respective 63 operational definitions, is presented in Goodman et al. (1996).

The PIL is used to create a Patient Impairment Profile (PIP) for a given patient, consisting of those impairments identified as the focus of treatment. For each cited impairment on the PIP, a severity rating is also provided on a four-point scale (i.e., 1 = *distressing*, 2 = *destabilizing*, 3 = *incapacitating*, and 4 = *imminently dangerous*). These severity ratings do not indicate how upsetting impairments are for a patient, but rather how much impairments compromise normal functioning. Goodman et al. (1996) divided the 63 impairments into *noncritical* and *critical* categories. Noncritical impairments are theorized to be those that do not have the potential to become incapacitating or imminently dangerous (e.g., altered sleep), and therefore should only receive severity ratings of 1 or 2. In contrast, critical impairments do have the potential to become incapacitating or life threatening (e.g., substance abuse), and thus can receive severity ratings of 1, 2, 3, or 4.

The PIL addresses limitations of the DSM-IV. Klewicki, Bjorck, Leucht, and Goodman (1998) note that its impairment terms are designed to be mutually exclusive without overlap. Moreover, because PIL impairments are more specific than DSM-IV diagnoses, there should be more homogeneity within impairment categories than within DSM-IV diagnostic categories (Goldfried & Wolfe, 1998). The PIL also includes a quantitative dimension (severity ratings) not found in most DSM-IV categories, even though the advantages of quantitative versus solely categorical measurement are acknowledged in DSM-IV (p. xxii). In addition, using the PIL to create a PIP facilitates treatment planning, because each listed impairment logically implies a treatment goal (i.e., repair or reduction to maintenance level of that impairment; Goodman et al., 1996). These goals, in turn, provide a basis for generating treatment objectives and interventions. Furthermore, the PIP documents progress over time, via changes in impairment severity ratings.

1570   *Journal of Clinical Psychology, December 1999*

If any nomenclature is to facilitate communication regarding patients' needs, reliability and validity must be demonstrated. Klewicki et al. (1998) evaluated the interrater and test-retest reliability of the PIL in a vignette study using 16 advanced graduate students from a clinical psychology doctoral program. Interrater consistency regarding individual PIL impairments was good to excellent, with median true positive ratings of 93.8% (range = 56.3%–100%) and median true negative ratings of 98.4% (range = 86.1%–100%). Interrater consistency (Cronbach's alpha) for the entire set of 63 impairments was .67 regarding the presence or absence of impairments and .86 regarding severity ratings for all impairments. Test-retest reliability (i.e., percent of agreement regarding the presence of individual impairments) for a random subsample of five raters was fair to good over a six-month interval (range = 40%–100%; median = 100).

Klewicki et al. (1998) also assessed content validity. Their qualitative analyses suggested that the 63 PIL impairments comprise a comprehensive nomenclature that is representative of and relevant to the domain of treatable mental health impairment (Nunnally & Bernstein, 1994). Content validity is also reflected by the accuracy, specificity, and clarity of a measure's items (Haynes, Richard, & Kubany, 1995). Toward this end, Klewicki et al.'s qualitative analyses of individual impairments revealed a relatively miniscule occurrence of either consistent false positives or false negatives.

It is also essential to examine the degree to which the PIL demonstrates the expected (theorized) relationships with established measures (Foster & Cone, 1995; Nunnally & Bernstein, 1994). Such construct validation is needed to support the assertions that the PIL can accurately describe patients' treatment needs and can inform treatment planning. Thus, the current study assessed construct validity by comparing the PIL to existing measures of psychiatric dysfunction.

Evaluating the entire PIL requires its application to cases manifesting the complete range of mental health impairments. This was accomplished by carefully constructing 20 prototypical analogue "patients," each portrayed in a separate vignette, who collectively depicted all 63 impairments. Previous research supports vignette use for psychometric assessment of diagnostic systems (e.g., Andersen & Hawthorn, 1989; Hasin & Link, 1988; Heumann & Morey, 1990; Hjortso, S., Butler, B., Clemmensen, L., Jepsen, P. W., Kastrup, M., Vilmar, T., & Bech, P., 1989; Knesper, Pagnucco, & Kalter, 1986; Marwit, 1996; Shepherd, Brooke, Cooper, & Lin, 1968; Sorensen, Hargreaves, & Frielander, 1982). Vignettes studies increase the standardization of validity assessment, with all raters examining identical clinical data. If such studies support the PIL's validity, it will then be appropriate to examine its application to actual cases. Given the low incidence of some patient dysfunctions, however, this would require hundreds—if not thousands—of patients to insure sufficient data to test each of the 63 impairments. Thus, whereas vignettes obviously limit generalizability of findings, their use represents a cost-effective primary evaluation of a classification system (Hjortso et al., 1989).

Hypotheses

A diagnostic system's construct validity can be assessed by comparing its clinical efficacy to that of an existing system. To do this, the current study compared the PIL with the DSM-III-R[2] regarding degree of rater accuracy in describing the 20 analogue patients. Given the specificity and exclusivity of PIL terms, we hypothesized that the true positive

---

[2] The purpose of the study was to compare the PIL to a familiar and well-established diagnostic system. Student raters were extensively trained in the use of the DSM-III-R, and the DSM-IV was in print for only several months prior to data collection. Thus, the former system was used when constructing vignettes for this study.

Appendix B: Empirical Research Articles   **241**

Patient Impairment Lexicon   *1571*

percentages for these terms would be better than true positive percentages for DSM-III-R diagnoses.

Construct validity is also supported if scores on a new measure correlate as theorized with scores on previously validated measures. Furthermore, a diagnostic system's validity is enhanced to the extent that its use is not adversely affected by variance among raters (e.g., their differing previous exposure to patients). Thus, we compared raters' PIL responses with their responses on an existing psychiatric measure and then examined this comparison again, after statistically controlling for variance in raters' past experience with actual patients. We predicted that overall PIL impairment severity ratings would correlate positively with overall impairment ratings produced by an established measure of psychiatric functioning. Moreover, these correlations were expected to remain significant even after controlling for effects of raters' past experience with patients and vignette imaginability.

Finally, we assessed the PIL's construct validity by testing the theoretically proposed division of impairments into noncritical and critical categories (Goodman et al., 1992). As described above, Goodman et al. proposed that 37 of the 63 impairments do not have the potential to be "incapacitating" or "imminently dangerous" and thus should only receive severity ratings of 1 or 2. Therefore, we assessed the severity ratings of impairments labeled by Goodman et al. as noncritical. In accordance with Goodman et al.'s model, noncritical impairments were anticipated to receive only noncritical (i.e., 1 or 2) versus critical (i.e., 3 or 4) severity ratings.

Method

Measures

Vignettes. Twenty vignettes described 20 identified patients, respectively, being seen for an initial clinical interview (see Appendix for an example vignette). Whereas vignettes often included multiple family members, only one person per vignette was identified as the patient. These identified patients ranged in age from 5 to 73 years ($M = 26.75$) and equally represented both genders and four ethnic groups (African American, Asian American, Caucasian, and Latino).[3] Vignettes were equally divided into five case types: (a) chronic adult, (b) acute adult, (c) child, (d) family, and (e) couple. They were each approximately one-page long, consisting of: (a) reason(s) for referral, (b) relevant history, (c) clinical presentation, and (d) assessment assumptions (e.g., no organicity was involved).

Each of Goodman et al.'s (1996) 63 impairments was present in at least one vignette.[4] Content validity of the vignettes was previously enhanced (Klewicki et al., 1998) through a series of revisions by four experts (a psychiatrist, a psychologist, and two clinical psychology graduate students) who used the following criteria: (a) imaginability, (b) inclusion of intended impairments, (c) exclusion of unintended impairments, and (d) inclusion of sufficient criteria for at least one DSM-III-R diagnosis per vignette. A variety of diagnoses were portrayed for the identified patients in these vignettes, such as schizophrenia, antisocial personality disorder, major depression, alcohol abuse, and encopresis (see Table 1).

---

[3] To minimize confounding variables, instructions included the assumption that all identified patients were fully fluent in English and completely acculturated to life within the United States. (Whereas ethnocultural variables merit direct investigation, they were beyond the current study's scope.)

[4] In order for all 20 identified patients to meet the criteria for a DSM-III-R diagnosis, it was necessary to depict seven impairments more than once. Altered sleep, egocentricity, and inadequate self-maintenance were each described in two of the 20 vignettes. Psychic agitation was described in three vignettes. Dysphoric mood and marital/relational dysfunction were each described in four vignettes, and family dysfunction was described in five vignettes. The remaining 58 impairments were each presented once.

Table 1

True Positive Reporting of Diagnoses (DSM-III-R) and Impairments (PII)

Vignette	Age/Gender/ Ethnicity	DSM-III-R Diagnoses	Averaged True Positives		PII Impairments
			DSM-II-R[a]	PII[b]	
1	35/Female/AA	Schizophrenia, Disorganized Type, Chronic with Acute Exacerbation	87.5	85.9	Delusions (Nonparanoid), Educational Performance Deficit, Inadequate Self-Maintenance Skills, Psychotic Thought/Behavior
2	24/Male/C	Schizophrenia, Paranoid Type, Chronic with Acute Exacerbation	93.8	89.1	Delusions (Paranoid), Hallucinations, Inadequate Health Care Skills, Inadequate Self-Maintenance Skills
3	41/Male/L	Antisocial Personality Disorder	100	78.1*	Assaultiveness, Fire Setting, Homicidal Thought/Behavior, Stealing
4	21/Female/AfA	Multiple Personality Disorder	68.8	96.9**	Alexithymia, Dissociative States, Mood Lability, Self-Mutilation
5	73/Male/AfA	Major Depression, Single Episode, Mild	43.8	95.3**	Altered Sleep, Concomitant Medical Condition, Dysphoric Mood, Medical Treatment Noncompliance
6	32/Male/C	Bipolar Disorder, Manic, Severe, without Psychotic Features	100	85.4	Manic Thought/Behavior, Medical Risk Factor, Uncontrolled Buying
7	47/Female/AfA	Obsessive-Compulsive Disorder	93.8	97.9	Compulsions, Obsessions, Psychic Agitation
8	24/Female/L	Alcohol Abuse	56.2	87.5**	Decreased Concentration, Psychomotor Retardation, Substance Abuse
9	7/Male/L	Post-Traumatic Stress Disorder	62.5	95.8**	Altered Sleep, Self-Esteem Deficiency, Sexual Trauma Victim
10	5/Male/AfA	Functional Enuresis, Nocturnal, Primary Type	100	75.0*	Enuresis, Pathological Guilt, Psychic Agitation

Patient Impairment Lexicon

			[a]	[b]	
11	9/Female/C	Attention-Deficit Hyperactivity Disorder, Moderate; Developmental Arithmetic Disorder; Functional Encopresis, Primary Type	70.8	83.3	Encopresis, Learning Disability, Motor Hyperactivity
12	15/Female/C	Bulimia Nervosa	100	93.8	Eating Disorder, Emotional Abuse Victim, Family Dysfunction, Physical Abuse Victim, Suicidal Thought/Behavior
13	40/Male/AfA	Pedophilia (Nonexclusive Type)	86.7	86.2	Emotional Abuse Perpetrator, Family Dysfunction, Marital/Relationship Dysfunction, Sexual Object Choice Dysfunction, Sexual Trauma Perpetrator
14	8/Male/L	Separation Anxiety Disorder	100	93.8	Family Dysfunction, School Avoidance, Somatization, Tantrums
15	14/Female/AfA	Major Depression, Single Episode, Moderate	37.5	81.2**	Dysphoric Mood, Family Dysfunction, Pathological Grief, Truancy
16	16/Female/AA	Oppositional Defiant Disorder, Moderate	93.8	95.3	Family Dysfunction, Lying, Oppositionalism, Running Away
17	30/Male/C	Pathological Gambling	93.8	95.0	Egocentricity, Marital/Relationship Dysfunction, Physical Abuse Perpetrator, Promiscuity, Uncontrollable Gambling
18	37/Female/L	Simple phobia	68.8	84.3	Dysphoric Mood, Phobia, Psychic Agitation, Social Withdrawal
19	28/Female/AA	Dysthymia, Histrionic Personality Disorder	59.4	90.0**	Dysphoric Mood, Egocentricity, Externalization/Blame, Manipulativeness, Marital/Relationship Dysfunction
20	29/Male/AA	Gender Identity Disorder Not Otherwise Specified, Male Erectile Disorder	46.9	85.9**	Gender Dysphoria, Marital/Relationship Dysfunction, Sexual Performance Dysfunction, Uncommunicativeness

[a] Numbers in this column are true positive percentages for the DSM-III-R diagnosis in each vignette, or the averaged true positive percentages in vignettes where there were multiple diagnoses.

[b] Numbers in this column are averaged true positive percentages for all impairments in each vignette.

*Significant two-tailed difference between diagnostic and impairment true positive percentages, $p < .05$.

**Significant two-tailed difference between diagnostic and impairment true positive percentages, $p < .01$.

Impairment inventory. To facilitate assessment of the PIL, a 63-item Patient Impairment Inventory (PII) was constructed based on Goodman et al.'s (1996) 63 impairment definitions. The inventory lists the impairments in two columns on an $8\frac{1}{2}''$ by $11''$ sheet of paper. Each impairment that applies to the patient is scored by the clinician on the four-point severity scale developed by Goodman et al. and ranging from 1 (*distressing*) to 4 (*imminently dangerous*). If an impairment does not apply to the patient, it is not marked. A separate inventory is used for each patient. For reference, raters were also provided with an $11''$ by $17''$ sheet listing Goodman et al's 63 impairments and their definitions, and a smaller ($8\frac{1}{2}''$ by $11''$) sheet listing definitions for the four impairment severity levels.[5] As described above, Klewicki et al.'s (1998) initial assessment of the interrater reliability of this instrument revealed moderate to high reliability of individual impairments and moderate reliability of the diagnostic system as a whole.

Similarity to past experience. The similarity of the 20 identified patients to real patients the raters had encountered previously was assessed with a one-item scale. This scale asks, "How *similar* was this case to *real* patients/clients you have actually interviewed in the past?" and ranges from 1 ("This case was extremely different than any case I have interviewed in the past") to 6 ("This case was very similar to a case I have interviewed in the past").

Vignette imaginability. As a manipulation check, imaginability of the vignettes was also rated with a one-item scale. This scale asked raters, "How *easy* was it for you to *imagine* yourself as the interviewer in the preceding vignette?" and ranges from 1 ("It was extremely difficult for me to do this") to 6 ("It was very easy for me to do this").

Psychiatric symptoms. Raters completed the Brief Psychiatric Rating Scale (BPRS; Overall & Gorham, 1962) for each identified patient. It consists of 16 clinician-rated items, each of which assesses a different symptom (e.g., somatic concerns, anxiety, depressive mood, disordered thoughts, bizarre behavior, hallucinations, etc.). The severity of each symptom is rated on a scale from 1 (*not present*) to 7 (*extremely severe*). A total pathology score is also computed by summing the individual item scores. Overall and Gorham found moderate interrater reliability for the individual items on the BPRS (range of $rs = .62–.87$). A more recent study of the BPRS found comparable interrater reliabilities for individual items ranging from .52 to .92 and a moderate total scale interrater reliability of .87 (Bell, Milstein, Beam-Goulet, Lysaker, & Cicchetti, 1992). The BPRS has been used widely in general, and has also specifically been used in recent studies attempting to establish concurrent validity of new psychiatric rating scales (e.g., Bell et al.; Manchanda, Saupe, & Hirsch, 1986).

Procedure

The data for the current study were collected as part of a larger research project involving the PIL. The 20 vignettes described above were administered in a group setting to 16 clinical psychology graduate students who were in either their fourth, fifth, or sixth year of study in a doctoral program. Raters were paid for their participation.

---

[5] Severity definitions were as follows: 1 = *Distressing*: Causes mental anguish or suffering in self/others; 2 = *Destabilizing*: Markedly weakens the ability to carry out daily activities and/or places self/others in potential danger; 3 = *Incapacitating*: Severely interferes with normal daily functioning and/or places self/others in likely danger; 4 = *Immanently Dangerous*: Immediately life-threatening to self/others (Goodman et al., 1996).

Appendix B: Empirical Research Articles   **245**

Patient Impairment Lexicon   *1575*

Before reading any vignettes, raters were given the following: (a) an impairment definition sheet and a severity-level definition sheet for the Patient Impairment Lexicon (described above), (b) two pages of detailed written instructions regarding measure completion, and (c) an example vignette with completed measures regarding its identified patient. Each rater also had a DSM-III-R manual for reference in assigning diagnoses. Raters were blind to the theorized division of impairments into noncritical and critical categories, in order to provide a better test of Goodman et al.'s (1992) model.

After reading the reference sheets, instructions, and example, raters were given booklets containing the 20 vignettes (in counterbalanced order) interleaved with 20 sets of the measures. Raters read each vignette and then: (a) completed a Patient Impairment Inventory for the identified patient, (b) provided appropriate DSM-III-R Axis I and/or Axis II diagnoses, (c) rated the imaginability of the vignette, (d) assessed the similarity of the identified patient to actual patients interviewed previously by the rater, and (e) completed a Brief Psychiatric Rating Scale.

While completing the measures, raters were to imagine that they had just conducted the clinical interview described in the vignette. They were also instructed to pay careful attention to the information given in the "Assessment Assumptions" section, and they were to assume that anything not mentioned in a given vignette had been ruled out. Thus, for each analog patient, data provided to raters approximated that which might be obtained via a structured interview.

Results

Descriptive Statistics

Table 1 presents the demographic information on the analog patients described in the 20 vignettes. Descriptive statistics were also calculated regarding the similarity of depicted analog patients to raters' actual past patients. Raters found the depicted patients to be only slightly similar ($M = 3.55$, $SD = .45$) to real patients they had seen previously. Thus, these graduate student raters' diagnostic experience might be underrepresentative compared to the general population of experienced expert clinicians. The average imaginability of vignettes was also calculated ($M = 4.49$, $SD = .59$), indicating that raters generally found the vignettes to be somewhat easy to imagine. Given that these vignettes depicted cases only slightly similar to their past experience, rater's imaginability ratings supported use of the vignettes.

Comparison of Interrater Accuracy

Table 1 also presents information related to the comparison of true positive percentages for diagnoses (DSM-III-R) and impairments (PII). Specifically, these percentages represent the degree to which raters correctly identified those diagnoses and impairments portrayed in each vignette. Some vignettes portrayed more than one diagnosis and all vignettes portrayed more than one impairment. Thus, percentages represent the true positive averages for each vignette. For impairments, Table 1 lists true positives concerning impairment type, without regard to severity ratings. To achieve parallel measurement precision, DSM-III-R true positives represent correct identification of diagnostic type, without regard to modifiers such as severity.

The overall average true positive percentage for the entire PII (across all 20 vignettes) was higher ($M = 88.8\%$, $SD = 6.4$) than the overall DSM diagnostic true positive percentage ($M = 78.2\%$, $SD = 20.8$) and this mean difference was significant, $F(1, 18) =$

1576   *Journal of Clinical Psychology, December 1999*

Table 2
Hierarchical Regression of Rater Number, Vignette Imaginability, Similarity of Experience, and PII Total Score on BPRS Total Scores

Variable	Effect Size	Sum of Squares	df_1	Mean Square	F Ratio	p
Rater Number	$\acute{\eta} = .47$	3945.01	15	263.00	6.83	<.0001
Vignette Imaginability	$r = .06$	71.85	1	71.85	1.87	=.2
Similarity of Experience	$r = .15$	413.73	1	413.73	10.75	<.005
PII Total Score	$r = .33$	1977.06	1	1977.06	51.36	<.0001

Note. $df_2 = 301$, $N = 320$. Tests have all prior independent variables partialled out. Effect size is product-moment correlation (r) or eta ($\acute{\eta}$) with prior variables partialled out. Tests are two-tailed.

4.48, $p < .05$. In addition, individual generalized likelihood ratio tests (Larsen & Marx, 1986) for each of the 20 vignettes showed that true positive percentages were significantly higher ($p < .05$ in all cases) for impairments than for diagnoses in seven vignettes (see Table 1). In contrast, significant findings contrary to expectations ($p < .05$) were only found for two vignettes (see Table 1).

Correlations with Established Measures

In order to compare the PIL to an established measure of psychiatric function it was first necessary to insure that scores from both were at a comparable level of aggregation (Rushton, Brainerd, & Pressley, 1983). The BPRS total score provides a global measure of psychopathology, including assessment of a wide range of symptoms (e.g., somatic concerns, anxiety, depressive mood, disordered thoughts, bizarre behavior, hallucinations, etc.). Thus, a global rating of psychiatric impairment severity based on the PIL was also needed for each patient. This was computed via the linear combination of each patient's PII severity scores, resulting in a PII total score. Technically, these total scores could range from zero (i.e., no impairments noted) to 252 (i.e., all 63 impairments cited and rated as 4 = imminently dangerous).

Two analyses were conducted to assess the correlation between the PII and the BPRS. First, for each of the 20 vignettes, the PII and BPRS total scores were respectively averaged across the 16 raters (to control for rater error), resulting in one pair of scores for each vignette. A significant correlation between these 20 PII scores and 20 BPRS scores was found, $r(1,18) = .45$, $p < .05$, one-tailed. Next, as a more conservative test of construct validity, the relationship between the PII and the BPRS was assessed again, controlling for variance due to raters, similarity of experience, and vignette imaginability. To accomplish this, each of the 16 raters' PII and BPRS scores for each of the 20 vignettes were considered as individual data points, resulting in 320 pairs of scores. Then, a hierarchical regression was conducted of rater number,[6] experience, imaginability, and PII scores on BPRS scores, using sequential sums of squares. Thus, the relationship between PII total scores and BPRS scores reflected unique variance. Table 2 shows that rater variance did significantly impact the ratings on both measures ($\eta = .47$). In addition, whereas vignette imaginability was not related to influence BPRS scores, raters' previous

---

[6]Gorsuch's (1991) statistical program *Unimult* uses a unified multivariate approach, incorporating generalized multiple correlation (η). This statistical design allows for the conjoint entry of nominal and continuous variables in multiple regression equations.

Appendix B: Empirical Research Articles   **247**

Patient Impairment Lexicon   *1577*

experience was ($r = .15$). After controlling for these three variables, however, the predicted positive relationship between PII and BPRS scores remained significantly positive ($r = .33, p < .0001$, two-tailed).

Severity Ratings for Noncritical Impairments

Next, the 37 proposed noncritical impairments (Goodman et al., 1992) were examined regarding the extent to which they actually received noncritical ratings of 1 or 2, in support of Goodman et al.'s model, versus critical ratings of 3 or 4. For each of these impairments, the percentage of raters who assigned severity ratings of 1 or 2 was calculated (see Table 3).Percentages ranged widely (11%–100%). Twenty-six of the 37 theorized noncritical impairments were rated as noncritical at least 66% of the times they were identified. Six impairments hypothesized to be noncritical were rated as noncritical less than 50% of the times they were rated (emotional abuse perpetrator, stealing, inadequate self-maintenance skills, uncontrolled gambling, promiscuity, and sexual object choice dysfunction).

Discussion

The present study contributed to the validation of the PIL first by comparing its clinical utility to that of the DSM-III-R. In support of hypotheses, comparing rater accuracy on PIL impairments to rater accuracy on DSM-III-R diagnoses revealed that raters' average true positive percentage was significantly higher for PIL impairments (88.8%) than for DSM-III-R diagnoses (78.2%). Furthermore, rater accuracy was significantly higher on impairments than diagnoses in seven individual vignettes. Whereas the reverse was true for two vignettes, these two depicted impairments (pathological guilt, fire setting) previously shown to have low reliabilities relative to the entire 63 impairments (Klewicki et al., 1998). Overall, raters were better able to correctly identify the presence or absence of an array of particular clinical impairments (e.g., dysphoric mood, hallucinations, tantrums, etc.) than they were able to differentially diagnose specific psychiatric disorders. This suggests that raters can agree on patients' impairments as much as, if not more than, patients' diagnoses. Such agreement among raters is crucial for standardized communication within MBHOs if mental health resources are to be disbursed fairly and consistently.

It is encouraging that a moderate to high level of impairment rating accuracy was found in a group of raters who had received minimal instruction in the use of the PIL (i.e., exposure to only one training example), whereas their DSM-III-R training had been extensive. This preliminary evidence suggests that the PIL is a system that can be learned relatively quickly and used immediately with a fair amount of accuracy. This is another highly desirable characteristic for a measure designed for use within MBHOs, because participants in these systems are often spread out over large distances and numerous settings (making universal training for participants more difficult), and because time and financial resources for staff training can be limited.

It is also noteworthy that in some vignettes, the correct impairments provided much more specific clinical information than the correct diagnosis did. For example, the correct DSM-III-R diagnosis for Vignette 17 was pathological gambling (see Table 1), whereas the correct Patient Impairment Profile for this vignette included egocentricity, marital/relationship dysfunction, physical abuse perpetrator, promiscuity, and uncontrollable gambling. Thus, a clinician developing a Patient Impairment Profile in conjunction with a diagnosis for this particular patient would be much closer to developing a comprehensive

Table 3

Average Percentages of Noncritical Severity Ratings
for Noncritical Impairments

Impairment	n[a]	% Noncritical Ratings[b]
Uncommunicativeness	16	100.0
Encopresis	15	93.3
Manipulativeness	15	93.3
Educational performance deficit	12	91.7
Altered sleep	30	90.0
Learning disability	10	90.0
Decreased concentration	15	86.7
Enuresis	15	86.7
Lying	15	86.7
Truancy	15	86.7
Gender dysphoria	15	80.0
Pathological grief	15	80.0
Externalization/blame	14	78.6
Tantrums	13	77.0
Medical treatment noncompliance	16	75.0
Self-esteem deficiency	16	75.0
Somatization	16	75.0
Marital/relationship dysfunction	59	74.6
Alexithymia	15	73.3
Emotional abuse victim	15	73.3
Pathological guilt	11	72.7
Egocentricity	30	70.0
Sexual performance dysfunction	16	68.8
Family dysfunction	66	68.2
Oppositionalism	15	66.7
Sexual trauma victim	15	66.7
Social withdrawal	14	64.3
Motor hyperactivity	15	60.0
Uncontrolled buying	15	60.0
School avoidance	16	56.2
Physical abuse victim	15	53.3
Emotional abuse perpetrator	15	46.7
Stealing	13	46.2
Inadequate self-maintenance skills	25	44.0
Uncontrolled gambling	16	31.2
Promiscuity	15	20.0
Sexual object choice dysfunction	9	11.1

[a]The number of times an impairment was rated could range from 1 to 16, for impairments presented only once, to 1 to 80 for an impairment depicted five times (i.e., Family Dysfunction).
[b]Noncritical percentages refer to the number of times that the given impairment was rated as noncritical out of the total number of times that the impairment was rated. Noncritical ratings supported the theorized model of impairments (Goodman, Brown, & Deitz, 1992), whereas critical ratings disconfirmed the theorized model.

treatment plan than if he or she had only determined the appropriate diagnosis. Likewise, a utilization reviewer who saw this patient's impairment profile and diagnosis would have a much better sense of why treatment is needed and what forms of treatment are indicated than if the reviewer only had access to the patient's diagnosis.

Another way in which the PIL was compared to existing measures was by examining its relationship to the BPRS. The sample size for correlating responses to these two

Appendix B: Empirical Research Articles

Patient Impairment Lexicon

measures, averaged across raters, was small ($N = 20$). Given the resulting very low statistical power, the fact that this correlation ($r = .45$) was significant is notable and supports the construct validity of the PIL. Still, the relationship between the PII scores and BPRS scores were potentially confounded by rater error, level of raters' past experience with patients, and vignette imaginability. Our second analysis showed that even after controlling for these confounds, however, the positive relationship between the PIL and the BPRS remained.

Finally, the theorized classification of impairments (i.e., noncritical versus critical) received poor to only modest support. This might have been partly due to our conservative methodology, which included not informing raters that noncritical impairments should theoretically only receive severity ratings of 1 or 2. As such, raters probably assumed that severity ratings of 1, 2, 3, or 4 were potentially applicable to all impairments, making errors more likely. Given this, the fact that 26 of the 37 theorized noncritical impairments were still rated as noncritical at least two-thirds of the time is somewhat encouraging. In contrast, six of the theorized noncritical impairments (emotional abuse perpetrator, stealing, inadequate self-maintenance skills, uncontrolled gambling, promiscuity, and sexual object choice dysfunction) received severity ratings of 1 or 2 (noncritical) less than 50% of the time. Raters' frequent use of critical severity ratings (3 or 4) for these six impairments might have been due to confusion regarding instructions. For example, raters might have erroneously used severities to rate how upsetting an impairment was *to* the patient, rather than how dangerous it was *for* the patient. Alternately, severity scores might have been erroneously inflated because raters focused on a patient's most severe impairment and overgeneralized, failing to assess whether each individual impairment was truly incapacitating or imminently dangerous. For example, in Vignette 1, inadequate self-maintenance skills might have received an erroneous severity score of 3 or 4 from some raters because the patient in this vignette (see Table 1) did exhibit imminently dangerous behaviors attributable to another impairment (delusions). Clearly, given these problematic preliminary findings regarding the critical/noncritical classification of impairments, further refinements (e.g., concerning the classification itself, clarification of instructions, etc.) are needed.

The current findings must be interpreted in light of methodological limitations. First, the utility of the PIL was assessed with ratings of patients depicted in vignettes rather than actual patients, and these depictions were only slightly similar to cases that raters had experienced previously. Whereas these factors probably reduced external validity, this is offset to some extent by the fact that vignettes were also rated as at least somewhat easy to imagine. Moreover, findings remained significant even after partialling out variance due to both experience and imaginability. Clearly, these preliminary findings support the need for clinical studies of the PIL, using real patient samples exhibiting the entire range of diagnoses. Second, the present study compared the PIL to DSM-III-R, and not to DSM-IV. This decision was justified by the fact that DSM-IV was only recently published when data was collected, whereas raters had extensive DSM-III-R training. Moreover, care was taken to employ DSM-III-R diagnostic categories that were not changed in major ways in DSM-IV. Future PIL research will obviously incorporate the DSM-IV. Third, given that the same raters provided both BPRS and PII scores, the correlations between these two measures might have been inflated. This was addressed by partialling out variance due to raters, but future research might also benefit from using different raters to obtain the two sets of scores. Finally, although an attempt was made to portray patients in the vignettes as being from various ethnic backgrounds and both genders, this does not in itself insure that PIL impairments will be understood and rated in a consistent way across cultural contexts. Future PIL research will need to assess the impact of factors such as gender, ethnicity, and culture.

Conclusion

Despite its limitations, the current study provides preliminary support for the construct validity of the PIL as a measure of psychiatric functioning. Current findings suggest that the PIL can augment diagnostic information and facilitate treatment planning, while specifically answering MBHOs' question, "Why is treatment needed?" Moreover, the PIL appears to be readily learned with minimal instruction. Future research clearly must replicate these findings with actual patients in studies with very large sample sizes. Recent developments have made the execution of such studies more feasible. Specifically, the PIL has now been incorporated in a comprehensive software product that automates its impairment-based documentation method (Community Sector Systems, 1997), making wide-scale centralized use (e.g., by MBHOs) of this system feasible. Such wide-scale use will permit the generation of clinically rich databases and enable continual empirical refinement of this system. Thus, in the ongoing efforts to optimize mental healthcare quality, the PIL is one clinical tool that holds promise.

Appendix

Case Presentation #5: "Vince"

Reason for Referral. Vince, a 73-year-old African-American male, was referred to you for evaluation by his physician. He is complaining of difficulty sleeping. In addition, his physician feels that he is having trouble getting used to his new treatment regimen. This concern is supported by his gradual but significant weight gain (15 lbs.) over the past eight weeks, following his being diagnosed with Late Onset Diabetes. Vince's sleeping difficulties also began after receiving this diagnosis. He complains of almost always having trouble falling asleep initially, and also after waking up to use the bathroom. He feels the sleep loss may explain why "I always feel drained." His physician states that Vince's diabetes is mild and can be controlled with oral medication. Still, the physician is concerned that Vince's "forgetting" (one to two times weekly) to take his daily pills could present a medical risk in the future, especially if his condition should worsen. You interview Vince, and obtain the following information:

History. Vince reports that he has "never been sick a day in my life" until the onset of his diabetes. He is "happily married" and enjoys spending time with his grandchildren. He states that receiving his diagnosis "made me face the fact that I am not getting any younger." For the last month, he has found himself continually "feeling blue" and preoccupied with morbid issues, especially at bedtime (e.g., death, estate planning, his own parents' deaths 15 and 17 years earlier, respectively). This in turn has made it hard to fall asleep. "Then I started waking up a lot too, to use the bathroom; but the doctor says I just have to get used to that as part of this awful disease." He describes his wife as "very supportive," but adds, "I don't like to bother her with this. She's got enough problems with her bad back." He further states, "I have always taken care of her, and it feels strange to have the shoe on the other foot."

Clinical Presentation. Vince presents as a well-dressed and groomed, obese male of average height. He appears calm and he attempts to be cheerful, but does become tearful at times. He is alert, articulate, maintains good eye contact, and is generally pleasant— even when recounting his current difficulties. When questioned, Vince admits, "I do forget those silly pills quite often." In addition, he admits that his forgetfulness "is probably due to my not wanting to accept this." He further explains that "life would be terrific

Appendix B: Empirical Research Articles

Patient Impairment Lexicon

if I just didn't have this disease to deal with. I know I should watch my weight, but a few sweets now and then help me feel better. I guess I should be thankful for having had such good health up until now, but I just can't seem to help being upset about all this."

Assessment Assumptions. Sleeping difficulties and weight gain are related to, but not caused by, medical condition. The psychiatric symptoms are not organic. There is no substance abuse.

INSTRUCTIONS

Please complete all the questions that follow with respect to this case regarding *VINCE ONLY*. Remember that information not mentioned should be assumed to be nonapplicable to this case. Assume that all symptoms and/or relevant information are reported in the case description.

References

American Psychiatric Association (1987). Diagnostic and statistical manual for mental disorders (3rd ed., rev.). Washington, DC: Author.

American Psychiatric Association (1994). Diagnostic and statistical manual for mental disorders (4th ed.). Washington, DC: Author.

Andersen, S.M., & Hawthorn, B.H. (1989). The diagnostic knowledge inventory: A measure of knowledge about psychiatric diagnosis. Journal of Clinical Psychology, 45, 999–1013.

Bell, M., Milstein, R., Beam-Goulet, J., Lysaker, P., & Cicchetti, D. (1992). The Positive and Negative Syndrome Scale and the Brief Psychiatric Rating Scale: Reliability, comparability, and predictive validity. Journal of Nervous and Mental Disease, 180, 723–728.

Calhoun, K.S., Moras, K., Pilkonis, P., & Rehm, L.P. (1998). Empirically supported treatments: Implications for training. Journal of Consulting and Clinical Psychology, 66, 151–162.

Chrisman, A.K., Lancaster, M., Ross, R., Ainsworth, T.L., Hemmings, K., & Shaffer, I.A. (1996). Towards a standard documentation for behavioral health. Journal of Practical Psychiatry and Behavioral Health, 2, 105–110.

Clark, L.A., Watson, D., & Reynolds, S. (1995). Diagnosis and classification of psychopathology: Challenges to the current system and future directions. Annual Review of Psychology, 46, 121–153.

Community Sector Systems (1997). PsychAccess Clinical Information System: Provider module user's manual, version 2.1. Seattle, WA: Author.

Follette, W.C., & Houts, A.C. (1996). Models of scientific progress and the role of theory in taxonomy development: A case study of the DSM. Journal of Consulting and Clinical Psychology, 64, 1120–1132.

Foster, S.L., & Cone, J.D. (1995). Validity issues in clinical assessment. Psychological Assessment, 7(3), 248–260.

Frances, A., First, M.B., & Pincus, H.A. (1995). DSM-IV guidebook. Washington, DC: American Psychiatric Press.

Goldfried, M.R., & Wolfe, B.E. (1998). Toward a more clinically valid approach to therapy research. Journal of Consulting and Clinical Psychology, 66, 143–150.

Goodman, M., Brown, J., & Deitz, P. (1992). Managing managed care: A mental health practitioner's survival guide. Washington, DC: American Psychiatric Press.

Goodman, M., Brown, J., & Deitz, P. (1996). Managing managed care: A mental health practitioner's survival guide. Washington, DC: American Psychiatric Press.

Gorsuch, R.L. (1991) Unimult for univariate and multivariate data analysis. Altadena, CA: Unimult.

Hamilton, M. (1960). A rating scale for depression. Journal of Neurology, Neurosurgery, and Psychiatry, 23, 56–62.

Hamilton, M. (1967). Development of a rating scale for primary depressive illness. British Journal of Social and Clinical Psychology, 6, 278–296.

Hasin, D., & Link, B. (1988). Age and recognition of depression: Implications for a cohort effect in major depression. Psychological Medicine, 18, 683–688.

Hayes, S.C., Wilson, K.G., Gifford, E.V., Follette, V.M., & Strosahl, K. (1996). Experiential avoidance and behavioral disorders: A functional dimensional approach to diagnosis and treatment. Journal of Consulting and Clinical Psychology, 64, 1152–1168.

Haynes, S.N., Richard, D.C.S., & Kubany, E.S. (1995). Content validity in psychological assessment: A functional approach to concepts and methods. Psychological Assessment, 7, 238–247.

Heumann, K.A., & Morey, L.C. (1990). Reliability of categorical and dimensional judgments of personality disorder. American Journal of Psychiatry, 147, 498–500.

Hjortso, S., Butler, B., Clemmensen, L., Jepsen, P.W., Kastrup, M., Vilmar, T., & Bech, P. (1989). The use of case vignettes in studies of interrater reliability of psychiatric target syndromes and diagnoses: A comparison of ICD-8, ICD-10, and DSM-III. Acta Psychiatrica Scandinavica, 80, 632–638.

Klewicki, L.L., Bjorck, J.P., Leucht, C.A., & Goodman, M. (1998). Patient impairment lexicon: A psychometric analysis. Psychological Reports, 83, 547–570.

Knesper, D.J., Pagnucco, D.J., & Kalter, N.M. (1986). Agreement on patient diagnosis, treatment, and referral across provider groups. Professional Psychology: Research and Practice, 17, 331–337.

Larsen, R.L., & Marx, L. (1986). An introduction to mathematical statistics and its applications (2nd ed.). Englewood Cliffs, NJ: Prentice-Hall.

Manchanda, R., Saupe, R., & Hirsch, S.R. (1986). Comparison between the Brief Psychiatric Rating Scale and the Manchester Scale for the rating of schizophrenic symptoms. Acta Psychiatrica Scandinavica, 74, 563–568.

Marwit, S.J. (1996). Reliability of diagnosing complicated grief: A preliminary investigation. Journal of Consulting and Clinical Psychology, 64, 563–568.

Newman, R. (1996). APA requests treatment criteria from MBHOs. Practitioner, 10, 7.

Nunnally, J.C., & Bernstein, I.H. (1994). Psychometric theory (3rd ed.). New York: McGraw-Hill.

Overall, J.E., & Gorham, D.R. (1962). The Brief Psychiatric Rating Scale. Psychological Reports, 10, 799–812.

Potts, M.K., Daniels, M., Burnam, M.A., & Wells, K.B. (1990). A structured interview version of the Hamilton Depression Rating Scale: Evidence of reliability and versatility of administration. Journal of Psychiatric Research, 24, 335–350.

Rushton, J., Brainerd, C., & Pressley, N. (1983). Behavioral development and construct validation: The principle of aggregation. Psychological Bulletin, 94, 18–38.

Sechrest, L., McKnight, P., & McKnight, K. (1996). Calibration of measures for psychotherapy outcome studies. American Psychologist, 51, 1065–1071.

Shepherd, M., Brooke, E.M., Cooper, J.E., & Lin, T. (1968). An experimental approach of psychiatric diagnosis. Acta Psychiatrica Scandinavica, 44 (Suppl. 201), 7–89.

Sorensen, J.L., Hargreaves, W.A., & Friedlander, S. (1982). Child global rating scales: Selecting a measure of patient functioning in a large mental health system. Evaluation and Program Planning, 5, 337–347.

Wulfurt, E., Greenway, D.E., & Dougher, M.J. (1996). A logical functional analysis of reinforcement-based disorders: Alcoholism and pedophilia. Journal of Consulting and Clinical Psychology, 64, 1140–1151.

References

American Psychiatric Association: Diagnostic and Statistical Manual of Mental Disorders, 4th Edition. Washington, DC, American Psychiatric Association, 1994

Barlow D: Health care policy, psychotherapy research, and the future of psychotherapy. Am Psychol 51:1050–1058, 1996

Burns GL, Patterson DR: Conduct problem behaviors in a stratified random sample of children and adolescents: new standardization data on the Eyberg Child Behavior Inventory. Psychological Assessment 2:391–397, 1990

Chrisman AK, Lancaster M, Ross R, et al: Towards a standard documentation for behavioral health. Journal of Practical Psychiatry and Behavioral Health 2:105–110, 1996

Fischer J, Corcoran K: Measures for Clinical Practice: A Sourcebook, Vol 1: Couples, Families, and Children. New York, Free Press, 1994a

Fischer J, Corcoran K: Measures for Clinical Practice: A Sourcebook, Vol 2: Adults. New York, Free Press, 1994b

Goodman M, Brown J, Deitz P: Managing Managed Care: A Mental Health Practitioner's Survival Guide. Washington, DC, American Psychiatric Press, 1992

Goodman M, Brown JA, Deitz PM: Managing Managed Care II: A Handbook for Mental Health Professionals, 2nd Edition. Washington, DC, American Psychiatric Press, 1996

Howard KI, Moras K, Brill PL, et al: Evaluation of psychotherapy: efficacy, effectiveness, and patient progress. Am Psychol 51:1059–1064, 1996

Hudson WW: The WALMYR Assessment Scales Scoring Manual. Tempe, AZ, WALMYR Publishing, 1992

Klewicki LL, Bjorck JP, Leucht CA, et al: Patient Impairment Lexicon: a psychometric analysis. Psychol Rep 83:547–570, 1998 [Reprinted in Appendix B of this book.]

Kovacs M: Children's Depression Inventory. Pittsburgh, PA, University of Pittsburgh, 1979

Leucht CA, Bjorck JP, Klewicki LL, et al: The Patient Impairment Lexicon: a validation study. J Clin Psychol 55:1–16, 1999 [Reprinted in Appendix B of this book.]

Newman FL, Tejeda MJ: The need for research that is designed to support decisions in the delivery of mental health services. Am Psychol 51:1040–1059, 1996

Newman R: APA requests treatment criteria from MBHOs. Practitioner 10:7, 1996

Nunnally JC, Bernstein IH: Psychometric Theory, 3rd Edition. New York, McGraw-Hill, 1994

Phares EJ, Erksine N: The measurement of selfism. Educational and Psychological Measurement 44:597–608, 1984

Radloff LS: The CES-D Scale: a self-report depression scale for research in the general population. Applied Psychological Measurement 1:385–401, 1977

Sanderson WC: Introduction to series on empirically validated psychological treatments. The Clinical Psychologist 47:9, 1994

Spanier GB: Measuring dyadic adjustment: new scales for assessing the quality of marriage and similar dyads. Journal of Marriage and the Family 38:15–28, 1976

Spielberger C: State-Trait Anxiety Inventory for Adults. Palo Alto, CA, Mind Garden, 1983

Index

A

Absent (severity rating), 38
Accepting responsibility, 108
Accreditation requirements, 2
Aftercare, 5
AIDS, 20, 22, 92
Alcohol abuse
case example for (Yolanda), 24
DSM-IV diagnostic criteria for, 200
Alexithymia, 48, 50
case example for (Tamara), 46
common errors for, 26
definition update for, 10
Altered Sleep, 38–39, 54, 56, 100, 102, 180
case examples
for Dean, 98
for Juan, 52
for Vince, 178
patient objectives for, 192
progress summary toward, 192
progress update toward, 189
American Psychiatric Association, 195
American Psychological Association, 195–196
Antisocial personality disorder, 69
case example for (Carlos), 64
DSM-IV diagnostic criteria for, 204
Anxiety, 10, 22, 82
case examples
for Billy, 80
for Shirley, 20
common errors for, 42, 54, 84, 124, 158
Appropriateness of care, xi, 4
Assaultiveness, 66, 68
case example for (Carlos), 64
common errors for, 76, 94
Assessment (assess, assessing), xi, 1, 3, 7, 69, 82,
102, 196
Attention-deficit/hyperactivity disorder
case example for (Hannah), 86
DSM-IV diagnostic criteria for, 206
Authorization, 130, 195. *See also* Treatment
authorization

B

Behavior-based patient dysfunction, xi
Behavior-based treatment terminology, 2–3
Behavioral evidence, 15, 72
Behavioral managed care, 2–3

Bipolar I disorder, single manic episode
case example for (Dean), 98
DSM-IV diagnostic criteria for, 208
Bulimia nervosa
case example for (Pam), 28
DSM-IV diagnostic criteria for, 201

C

Cafeteria-style lists, 3
Case managers (case management), 2
Case presentations, 16, 20, 24, 28, 32, 40, 46, 52, 58,
64, 74, 80, 86, 92, 98, 110, 122, 138, 156, 178
April: schizophrenia, disorganized type, 74
discharge summary for, 171–173, 174
documenting treatment course for, 170
DSM-IV diagnostic criteria for, 205
Impairment Inventory for, 76
Patient Impairment Profile (PIP) for, 78, 104,
133, 151, 171
patient objectives for, 105–106, 133
progress update toward, 151–153
practitioner interventions for, 133–134
tracking progress for, 150, 151–153
treatment goals for, 104–105, 107
Billy: enuresis, nocturnal only, 80
discharge summary for, 175–176
documenting treatment course for, 174
DSM-IV diagnostic criteria for, 205
Impairment Inventory for, 82
Patient Impairment Profile (PIP) for, 84, 107,
135, 154, 175
patient objectives for, 107–108
progress update toward, 154–155
practitioner interventions for, 136
tracking progress for, 153–155
treatment goals for, 107–108
Carlos: antisocial personality disorder, 64
DSM-IV diagnostic criteria for, 204
Impairment Inventory for, 66, 68
Dean: bipolar I disorder, single manic episode, 98
DSM-IV diagnostic criteria for, 208
Impairment Inventory for, 100
Patient Impairment Profile (PIP) for, 102
Eddie: separation anxiety disorder, 122
DSM-IV diagnostic criteria for, 210
Impairment Inventory for, 124
Patient Impairment Profile (PIP) for, 126
patient objectives for, 127–128
treatment goals for, 127

255

Case presentations *(continued)*
    Frank: schizophrenia, paranoid type, 16
        DSM-IV diagnostic criteria for, 199
        Impairment Inventory for, 18
    George: pedophilia, sexually attracted to both, 32
        DSM-IV diagnostic criteria for, 201
        Impairment Inventory for, 34
    Hannah: attention-deficit/hyperactivity disorder;
            encopresis; mathematics disorder, 86
        DSM-IV diagnostic criteria for, 206
        Impairment Inventory for, 88
        Patient Impairment Profile (PIP) for, 90
    Inez: specific phobia, 156
        DSM-IV diagnostic criteria for, 211
        Impairment Inventory for, 158
        Patient Impairment Profile (PIP) for, 160–161,
            165
        patient objectives for, 161–162
            progress update toward, 165–166
        practitioner interventions for, 163
        tracking progress for, 164, 165–166
    Juan: posttraumatic stress disorder, 52
        DSM-IV diagnostic criteria for, 203
        Impairment Inventory for, 54, 56
    Karen: oppositional defiant disorder, 138
        DSM-IV diagnostic criteria for, 210
        Impairment Inventory for, 140
        Patient Impairment Profile (PIP) for, 142–143
        patient objectives for, 143–144
        practitioner interventions for, 145–146
    Lilly: dysthymic disorder; histrionic personality
            disorder, 110
        DSM-IV diagnostic criteria for, 209
        Impairment Inventory for, 112
        Patient Impairment Profile (PIP) for, 114, 116
        patient objectives for, 116–118
        treatment goals for, 116
    Mark: gender identity disorder, 40
        DSM-IV diagnostic criteria for, 202
        Impairment Inventory for, 42, 44
    Pam: bulimia nervosa, 28
        DSM-IV diagnostic criteria for, 201
        Impairment Inventory for, 30
    Shirley: obsessive-compulsive disorder, 20
        DSM-IV diagnostic criteria for, 200
        Impairment Inventory for, 22
    Tamara: dissociative identity disorder, 46
        DSM-IV diagnostic criteria for, 202
        Impairment Inventory for, 48, 50
    Vince: major depression, single episode, mild, 178
        discharge summary for, 190–192
        documenting treatment course for, 189–190
        DSM-IV diagnostic criteria for, 212
        Impairment Inventory for, 180
        Patient Impairment Profile (PIP) for, 182–183,
            187, 191
        patient objectives for, 183–184
            progress update toward, 188–189
        practitioner interventions for, 185
        tracking progress for, 186–189
        treatment goals for, 183

    Wanda: major depression, single episode,
            moderate, 58
        DSM-IV diagnostic criteria for, 204
        Impairment Inventory for, 60, 62
    Yolanda: alcohol abuse, 24
        DSM-IV diagnostic criteria for, 200
        Impairment Inventory for, 26
    Zack: pathological gambling; narcissistic traits,
            92
        DSM-IV diagnostic criteria for, 207
        Impairment Inventory for, 94
        Patient Impairment Profile (PIP) for, 96
Center for Epidemiologic Studies—Depressed Mood
        Scale, 178, 180, 183, 188, 191
Child Protective Services, 52
Children's Depression Inventory, 58
Chronicity, 56
Clinical necessity, 38
    definition of, 37
Clinical rationale, xi, 3–4, 38, 72, 140, 160
    definition of, 37
Common errors, 9, 18, 22, 26, 30, 34, 42, 44, 48, 50,
        54, 56, 60, 62, 66, 68, 76, 78, 82, 84, 88, 90,
        94, 96–97, 100, 102, 112, 114, 124, 126,
        140, 142, 158, 160, 180, 182
Common language, xi–xii, 3–4
Communication, 2, 4, 6, 15, 94, 100, 134, 196
Community Sector Systems (CSS), xii–xiii
Compulsions, 22
    case example for (Shirley), 20
Concomitant Medical Condition, 180, 182
    case example for (Vince), 178
    common errors for, 82, 182
    patient objectives for, 184
        patient summary toward, 192
        patient update toward, 188
    practitioner interventions for, 185
Content validity, 8
Contextual factors, 7
Cost-effectiveness, 197
Critical impairments, 4, 39, 44, 72, 142
    definition of, 37
Critical *vs.* noncritical impairments, 39, 72

D
Data, 2–3, 197
Decreased concentration, 26
    case example for (Yolanda), 24
    common errors for, 60, 88
Definition updates, 10–11
    Alexithymia, 10
    Delusions, 10
    Egocentricity, 10
    Hallucinations, 10
    Lying, 10
    Manic Thought/Behavior, 10
    Marital/Relationship Dysfunction With
            Substance Abuse, 10
    Motor Hyperactivity, 10
    Oppositionalism, 10

Index

Physical Abuse Victim, 10
Psychotic Thought/Behavior, 10
School Avoidance, 10
Self-Mutilation, 10
Tantrums, 10
Treatment goal, 11
Uncommunicativeness, 10
Definitions, 13, 37, 71, 103, 131, 149, 169.
    See also Operational definitions
Delusions, 7–8, 78
    definition update for, 10
Delusions (Nonparanoid), 76, 78
    case example for (April), 74
    common errors for, 22, 48
    patient objectives for, 105–106
        progress summary toward,
            172–173
        progress update toward, 151–152
    practitioner interventions for, 133
Delusions (Paranoid), 18
    case example for (Frank), 16
Demographics, 196
Destabilizing (severity rating), 38
Diabetes, 178, 182, 186, 190, 194
Diagnosis, xi, 3–4, 6, 9, 15, 194, 196–197.
    See also DSM-IV
    definition of, 13
Diagnostic criteria. *See* DSM-IV
Discharge plan, 4–5, 132
    definition of, 131
    including in treatment plan, 5
Discharge summary, 9
    for April: schizophrenia, disorganized type,
        171–174
    for Billy: enuresis nocturnal only, 175–176
    for Vince: major depression, single episode, mild,
        190
Disorder, 3
Dissociative identity disorder
    case example for (Tamara), 46
    DSM-IV diagnostic criteria for, 202
Dissociative states, 48, 50
    case example for (Tamara), 46
    common errors for, 50
Distressing (severity rating), 38
Division of Clinical Psychology (Division 12) of the
    American Psychological Association,
    195–196
Documentation, xi, 2, 5, 11, 196
DSM-IV, xi, 9, 15, 195, 197
    diagnosis, 3, 9, 69, 194
    diagnostic criteria, 6
        for April: schizophrenia, disorganized type,
          205
        for Billy: enuresis, nocturnal only, 205
        for Carlos: antisocial personality disorder, 204
        for Dean: bipolar I disorder; single manic
          episode, 208
        for Eddie: separation anxiety disorder, 210
        for Frank: schizophrenia, paranoid type, 199

for George: pedophilia, sexually attracted to
    both, 201
for Hannah: attention-deficit/hyperactivity
    disorder; encopresis; mathematics
    disorder, 206
for Inez: specific phobia, 211
for Juan: posttraumatic stress disorder, 203
for Karen: oppositional defiant disorder, 210
for Lilly: dysthymic disorder; histrionic
    personality disorder, 209
for Mark: gender identity disorder, 202
for Pam: bulimia nervosa, 201
for Shirley: obsessive-compulsive disorder,
    200
for Tamara: dissociative identity disorder, 202
for Vince: major depression, single episode,
    mild, 212
for Wanda: major depression, single episode,
    moderate, 204
for Yolanda: alcohol abuse, 200
for Zack: pathological gambling; narcissistic
    traits, 207
Dyadic Adjustment Scale, 92
Dysphoric mood, 38–39, 60, 62, 112, 114, 158, 160,
    180, 182
    case examples
        for Inez, 156
        for Lilly, 110
        for Vince, 178
        for Wanda, 58
    common errors for, 26, 42, 48, 82, 160
    patient objectives for, 116, 183
        progress summary toward, 191
        progress update toward, 165–166
    practitioner interventions for, 163, 185
Dysthymic disorder
    case example for (Lilly), 110
    DSM-IV diagnostic criteria for, 209

E

Eating Disorder, 30
    case example for (Pam), 28
    common errors for, 180
Educational Performance Deficit, 39, 76, 78
    case example for (April), 74
    common errors for, 88
    patient objectives for, 106
        progress summary toward, 172–174
        progress update toward, 153
    practitioner interventions for, 134
Egocentricity, 7, 66, 68, 94, 96, 112, 114
    case examples
        for Carlos, 64
        for Lilly, 110
        for Zack, 92
    common errors for, 68, 100
    definition update for, 10
    patient objectives for, 117
Electronic claims, 196
Electronic information management, 196

Emotional Abuse Perpetrator
case example for (George), 32
Emotional Abuse Victim, 6, 30, 54, 56
case examples
for Juan, 52
for Pam, 28
Employee Assistance Program, 24
Encopresis, 88, 90, 206
case example for (Hannah), 86
common errors for, 90
Enuresis (impairment term), 82, 84
case example for (Billy), 80
patient objectives for, 107–108
progress summary toward, 176
progress update toward, 154
practitioner interventions for, 136
Enuresis, nocturnal only (diagnosis)
case example for (Billy), 80
DSM-IV diagnostic criteria for, 205
External review, xi
Externalization and Blame, 112, 114
case example for (Lilly), 110
common errors for, 34, 66
patient objectives for, 117
Extrapyramidal side effects, 74, 132, 150
Eyberg Child Behavior Inventory, 122, 124, 138

F

Family Dysfunction, 6–7, 30, 34, 60, 62, 72, 124,
140, 142
case examples
for Eddie, 122
for George, 32
for Karen, 138
for Pam, 28
for Wanda, 58
common errors for, 126
patient objectives for, 144
practitioner interventions for, 146
Fire setting, 66, 68
case example for (Carlos), 64

G

Gender dysphoria, 42
case example for (Mark), 40
common errors for, 44
Gender identity disorder
case example for (Mark), 40
DSM-IV diagnostic criteria for, 202
Goals and objectives, xi, 8, 103–130, 143, 148, 161,
174, 183, 196. *See also* Patient objectives;
Treatment goals

H

Haldol (haloperidol), 74, 132, 150
Hallucinations, 18
case example for (Frank), 16
definition update for, 10
Healthcare costs, xi

Health histories, 196
Histrionic personality disorder
case example for (Lilly), 110
DSM-IV diagnostic criteria for, 209
Homicidal Thought/Behavior, 66, 68
case example for (Carlos), 64

I

Identified patient, 15
Imipramine, 136
Impairment Inventory, 3, 9, 15, 69, 182
definition of, 13
Impairment Lexicon, xi–xiii, 7, 15, 100, 120, 140,
195, 197
definition of, 13
Impairments, 3–4, 39, 69, 72, 182, 194, 196
common language, 3
critical, 4, 39, 44, 72, 142
definition of, 37
definition of, 3, 13
noncritical, 4, 39, 72, 142
prioritization of, 72, 90, 94, 97, 126
repair of, 11, 104–105, 107
severity ratings of, xii, 4, 37–39, 62, 160
Inadequate Healthcare Skills, 18
case example for (Frank), 16
Inadequate Self-Maintenance Skills, 18, 76, 78
case examples
for April, 74
for Frank, 16
common errors for, 112
patient objectives for, 106
progress summary toward, 173
progress update toward, 152
practitioner interventions for, 134
Interrater reliability, xi. *See also* Reliability
Interventions, 1, 8–9, 132, 146, 148, 196.
See also Practitioner interventions
definition of, 5, 131

L

Learning Disability, 88, 90
case example for (Hannah), 86
common errors for, 76
Level of care, 2, 11, 38, 72, 155
definition of, 71
Lithium, 98, 100
Lying, 140, 142
case example for (Karen), 138
common errors for, 34, 94
definition update for, 10
patient objectives for, 144
practitioner interventions for, 146

M

Major depression, 6, 15
single episode, mild
case example for (Vince), 178
DSM-IV diagnostic criteria for,
212

Index

single episode, moderate
    case example for (Wanda), 58
    DSM-IV diagnostic criteria for, 204
Managed behavioral care organizations, xii, 194, 196
Managed care, xi, xiii
  definition of, 2
Manic Thought/Behavior, 100, 102
    case example for (Dean), 98
    definition update for, 10
Manipulativeness, 112
    case example for (Lilly), 110
    common errors for, 124
Marital/Relationship Dysfunction, 6, 11, 34, 42, 94, 96, 112, 114
    case examples
      for George, 32
      for Lilly, 110
      for Mark, 40
      for Zack, 92
    common errors for, 66, 96–97, 114, 140
    patient objectives for, 118
Marital/Relationship Dysfunction With Substance Abuse
    definition update for, 10
Mathematics disorder
    case example for (Hannah), 86
    DSM-IV diagnostic criteria for, 206
Medicaid, 2
Medical records, xi
Medical Risk Factor, 100, 102
    case example for (Dean), 98
    common errors for, 30, 180
Medical Treatments Noncompliance, 180, 182
    case example for (Vince), 178
    common errors for, 18
    patient objectives for, 184
      progress summary toward, 192
      progress update toward, 188–189
    practitioner interventions for, 185
Medicare, 2, 196
Mental (or behavioral) healthcare, 1–2
Methodological limitations, 197
Mood Lability, 48, 50
    case example for (Tamara), 46
    common errors for, 112
Motor Hyperactivity, 88, 90
    case example for (Hannah), 86
    common errors for, 100
    definition update for, 10
Multidisciplinary treatment, 196

N

Narcissistic traits
    case example for (Zack), 92
    DSM-IV diagnostic criteria for, 207
Necessitate and justify care, 3
No-suicide contract, 8
Nomenclature, 6. *See also* Impairment Lexicon
Noncritical impairments, 4, 39, 72, 142
Noncritical *vs.* critical impairments, 39, 72

O

Objectives, xi, 8, 130, 194. *See also* treatment objectives
Obsessions, 22
    case example for (Shirley), 20
    common errors for, 18, 158
Obsessive-compulsive disorder
    case example for (Shirley), 20
    DSM-IV diagnostic criteria for, 200
Operational definitions, 7–8, 15, 78, 82, 94, 100, 140
  modifications of, 10
Operationally defined terminology, 8
Oppositional defiant disorder
    case example for (Karen), 138
    DSM-IV diagnostic criteria for, 210
Oppositionalism, 7, 140, 142
    case example for (Karen), 138
    common errors for, 142
    definition update for, 10
    patient objectives for, 144
    practitioner interventions for, 146
Organic psychiatric symptoms, 15
Outcome, xii, 2, 170, 196
  definition of, 169
Outcome measure, 2, 104
  definition of, 103

P

Pathological gambling
    case example for (Zack), 92
    DSM-IV diagnostic criteria for, 207
Pathological grief, 60, 62
    case example for (Wanda), 58
    common errors for, 62
Pathological guilt, 82, 84
    case example for (Billy), 80
    patient objectives for, 108
      progress summary toward, 176
      progress update toward, 155
    practitioner interventions for, 136
Patient dysfunction, 15, 68–69
Patient Impairment Profile (PIP), xi–xii, 3, 5–6, 8–9, 15, 69, 196
  definition of, 71
  for April: schizophrenia, disorganized type, 78, 104, 133, 151, 171
  for Billy: enuresis, nocturnal only, 84, 107, 135, 154, 175
  for Eddie: separation anxiety disorder, 126–127
  for Hannah: attention-deficit/hyperactivity disorder; encopresis; mathematics disorder, 90
  for Inez: specific phobia, 160–161, 165
  for Karen: oppositional defiant disorder, 142–143
  for Lilly: dysthymic disorder; histrionic personality disorder, 114, 116
  for Vince: major depression, single episode, mild, 182–183, 187, 191
  for Zack: pathological gambling; narcissistic traits, 96

Patient objectives, xii, 4–5, 9, 104
    definition of, 5, 103
    for specific impairments
        concomitant medical condition, 184
        delusions (nonparanoid), 105–106, 151–152
        dysphoric mood, 116, 162, 183, 185
        educational performance deficit, 106, 153
        egocentricity, 117
        enuresis, 107–108
        externalization and blame, 117
        family dysfunction, 144
        inadequate self-maintenance skills, 106, 152
        lying, 144
        marital/relationship dysfunction, 118
        medical treatments noncompliance, 184
        oppositionalism, 144
        pathological guilt, 108
        phobia, 161
        psychotic thought/behavior, 105–106, 151–152
        running away, 143
        school avoidance, 128
        social withdrawal, 162
        somatization, 128
        tantrums, 127
    progress summary toward, 172–173, 176, 191–192
    progress update toward, 151–155, 165–166, 188–189
    target objectives, 104, 153
        definition of, 103
Patient outcome. See also Outcome
    definition of, 169
Patient problems, 3
Patient progress, xii, 9, 104, 149–168
Pedophilia, sexually attracted to both
    case example for (George), 32
    DSM-IV diagnostic criteria for, 201
Performance measures, 3
    definition of, 149
Personality traits, 7
Phobia, 158, 160
    case example for (Inez), 156
    common errors, 22
    patient objectives for, 161
        progress update toward, 165
    practitioner interventions for, 163
Physical Abuse Perpetrator
    case example for (Zack), 92
Physical Abuse Victim, 6, 30, 56
    case example for (Pam), 28
    definition update for, 10
Posttraumatic stress disorder
    case example for (Juan), 52
    DSM-IV diagnostic criteria for, 203
Practice guidelines, 2, 195, 197
Practitioner interventions, xii, 4
    definition of, 5
    for concomitant medical condition, 185
    for delusions (nonparanoid), 133
    for dysphoric mood, 163, 185
    for educational performance deficit, 134
    for enuresis, 136

    for family dysfunction, 146
    for inadequate self-maintenance skills, 134
    for lying, 146
    for medical treatment noncompliance, 134, 185
    for oppositionalism, 146
    for pathological guilt, 136
    for phobia, 163
    for psychotic thought/behavior, 134
    for running away, 145
    for social withdrawal, 163
Preauthorization of treatment, 2
Preferred provider, xi
Prioritizing impairments, 72, 90, 97, 126
Private practice, 2
Problem lists, 3
Process of care
    definition of, 149
Progress. See Patient progress
Promiscuity, 94, 96
    case example for (Zack), 92
Prozac (fluoxetine), 116, 184, 186, 190
Psychometric research, xi, xiii, 10, 196
Psychomotor Retardation
    case example for (Yolanda), 24
Psychotic Thought/Behavior, 7–8, 72, 76, 78
    case example for (April), 74
    common errors for, 18, 78
    definition update for, 10
    patient objectives for, 105–106
        progress summary toward, 172–173
        progress update toward, 151–152
    practitioner interventions for, 134

Q
Quality standards, 3

R
Rationale for recommended treatments, 2
Raynaud's disease, 98, 100
Reason for referral, 15
Recidivism, 197
Reimbursement, xi, 2
Reliability, 9–11, 15, 78, 94, 100, 104, 195–196
    interrater, xi
Reliable, 8. See also Valid
Repair of an impairment, 11, 104, 107, 120
Restoril (temazepam), 186–187
Reviewers, 2. See also Case managers
Risperdal (risperidone), 132–134, 150
Running away, 140, 142
    case example for (Karen), 138
    patient objectives for, 143
    practitioner interventions for, 145

S
Schizophrenia
    disorganized type
        case example for (April), 74
        DSM-IV diagnostic criteria for, 205

Index   **261**

paranoid type
    case example for (Frank), 16
    DSM-IV diagnostic criteria for, 199
School Avoidance, 7, 124, 126
    case example for (Eddie), 122
    common errors for, 60
    definition update for, 10
    patient objectives for, 128
Self-blame, 108
Self-care, 5, 38, 44
Self-Esteem Deficiency, 54, 56
    case example for (Juan), 52
    common errors for, 30, 56
Self-Mutilation, 48, 50
    case example for (Tamara), 46
    common errors for, 50
    definition update for, 10
Separation anxiety disorder
    case example for (Eddie), 122
    DSM-IV diagnostic criteria for, 210
Severely incapacitating (severity rating), 38
Severities, 39, 44, 72, 120, 196. *See also* Severity
    ratings
Severity ratings (severities), xii, 4, 9, 39, 62, 72, 90,
    160, 168
    definition of, 4, 37
Sexual Object Choice Dysfunction, 34
    case example for (George), 32
Sexual Performance Dysfunction
    case example for (Mark), 40
    common errors for, 44
Sexual Trauma Perpetrator, 34
    case example for (George), 32
Sexual Trauma Victim
    case example for (Juan), 52
    common errors for, 56
Social Withdrawal, 158, 160
    case example for (Inez), 156
    common errors for, 26
    patient objectives for, 162
        progress update toward, 166
    practitioner interventions for, 163
Software, xii, 2, 196
Somatization, 124, 126
    case example for (Eddie), 122
    patient objectives for, 128
Specific phobia
    case example for (Inez), 156
    DSM-IV diagnostic criteria for, 211
Standardized measures, 150, 168
Standardized treatment documentation, 2
State-Trait Anxiety Inventory for Adults, 156, 158,
    161, 165
Stealing, 66, 68
    case example for (Carlos), 64
Stuffing inventories, 39
Substance Abuse, 11, 26
    case example for (Yolanda), 24
Suicidal Thought/Behavior, 30
    case example for (Pam), 28
Suicide, contract prohibiting, 8

T

Tantrums, 72, 124, 126
    case example for (Eddie), 122
    common errors for, 140
    definition update for, 10
    patient objectives for, 127
Target objective, 104, 153. *See also* Patient objectives
    definition of, 103
Task Force on the Promotion and Dissemination of
    Psychological Procedures of the American
    Psychological Association, 195–196
Theoretical orientation, 5
Third-party payers, 195–196
Treatment authorization, xi. *See also* Authorization
Treatment durations, 196
Treatment efficacy, 197
Treatment endpoint, 11, 104
Treatment foci, 69, 72, 97
Treatment frequencies, 196
Treatment goals, 4–5, 9, 11, 104, 107–108, 116, 127
    definition of, 103, 120
    definition update for, 11
    endpoint goals, 11, 103–104, 107, 120, 135, 155,
        174, 183, 194
    interim goals, 11, 103–104, 120, 194
    maintenance goals, 11, 103–104, 107, 120, 130,
        174, 194
Treatment modality, 126, 132, 135, 146, 196
    definition of, 131
Treatment necessity, 4
Treatment plan, 3–5, 8, 131–148, 150, 165–166, 174,
    196. *See also* Practitioner interventions
    definition of, 131
    multidisciplinary treatment, 196
Treatment planning model, 4
Treatment settings, 4, 104, 196
Tricyclics, 184
Truancy, 60, 62
    case example for (Wanda), 58

U

Uncommunicativeness, 42
    case example for (Mark), 40
    common errors for, 54
    definition update for, 10
Uncontrolled buying, 100
    case example for (Dean), 98
    common errors for, 102
Uncontrolled gambling, 94, 96
    case example for (Zack), 92
Utilization criteria, 3

V

Valid, 8. *See also* Reliability
Validity, 15, 104, 195–196
Vignettes, 8. *See also* Case presentations